Say NO To Arthritis

Say no to ARTHRITIS

Patrick Holford

ION PRESS

Published by ION Press
5 Jerdan Place, London SW6 1BE
Tel: 071-385 7984
Fax: 071-385 3249

First published 1993

Cover design and illustrations: Christopher Quayle
Layout: Heather James

ISBN 1 870976 09 6

Printed in Great Britain by The Bath Press, Avon

CONTENTS

continued overleaf

GUIDE TO ABBREVIATED MEASURES

1 gram (g) = 1,000 milligrams (mg) = 1,000,000 micrograms (mcg)
Most vitamins are measured in milligrams or micrograms. Vitamins
A, D and E are also measured in International Units (iu), a
measurement designed to provide standardisation of the different
forms of these vitamins that have different potencies.

1mcg of retinol or 2mcg of beta carotene = 3.3iu of vitamin A
1mcg of vitamin D = 40iu
1mg of vitamin E = approx. 1iu of d-alpha tocopherol
1 pound (lb) = 16 ounces (oz)   2.2lbs = 1 kilogram (kg)
In this book calories means kilocalories (kcals)

2 teaspoons (tsp) = 1 dessertspoon (dsp)
3 teaspoons (tsp) = 1 tablespoon (tbsp)
1.5 dessertspoons = 1 tablespoon (tbsp)
5 ml = 1 teaspoon
10 ml = 1 dessertspoon
15 ml = 1 tablespoon

HOW TO USE THIS BOOK

Arthritis is not a single disease. There are many different kinds of arthritis, as well as associated conditions which are not technically called arthritis. This book aims to give you guidance on natural approaches to all kinds of arthritis and associated conditions.

THE INTRODUCTION helps you to identify what kind of arthritis you have. It also introduces you to the basic information, for example, what joints are made of, how healthy joints work, and how arthritis progresses, to enable you to understand more clearly the basis behind different approaches to the treatment of arthritis.

PART ONE helps you to identify the possible risk factors that can contribute to the development of arthritis, helping you to prevent further problems. It also covers new theories about the cause of and research into the treatment of arthritis.

PART TWO covers dietary approaches to arthritis, explaining the background to the Anti-Arthritis Diet recommended in this book.

PART THREE looks at the role vitamins and minerals play in arthritis, giving you the background to the recommendations to take specific dietary supplements.

PART FOUR examines physical and psychological aspects of arthritis to give you the basis behind, and the indications for, certain recommended exercises.

PART FIVE tells you what you actually need to do to help your body heal itself. This is the 'practical', not the 'theory'. So, if you've had enough of theory and research you can turn to PART FIVE and get on with it!

THE GLOSSARY on pages 152 to 153 explains medical terms referred to in the book, which are printed in italics the first time they occur.

INTRODUCTION

Why suffer?

Recently I had a call from a client I hadn't seen in several years. "What you recommended sorted out my arthritis, but now the symptoms are beginning to return" she told me. A simple diet and some supplements, based on a new way of looking at arthritis, kept her pain-free for seven years.

Arthritis is not an inevitable consequence of ageing, although in Britain nine in every ten people have it by the age of 60. But why do one in ten never develop arthritis? Why, in some communities, do nine in ten never develop arthritis? Arthritis, which means inflammation (itis) of a joint (athron), a term I use loosely here to describe a whole host of problems affecting joints, bones and muscles, is not simply a 'wear and tear' degenerative disease that is unavoidable. For example, in some African communities, whose people spend hours every day walking *without* shoes, arthritis is exceedingly rare.

When you consider that your body is the very latest model, shaped over millions of years of evolution, designed to deliver at least one hundred years of healthful living, should you accept that, when a part starts misbehaving, there is nothing you can do except dull the pain?

Arthritis starts with joint aches and pains. Many people put up with these early warning signs, until they develop into something a little more persistent. Then, a visit to the doctor may result in a prescription for an anti-inflammatory or pain-killing drug. Conventional drug treatments do nothing to cure the disease. At best, they reduce the pain. At worst, they speed up the progression of the disease. Severe arthritis is living hell and is probably responsible for more suffering than any other disease, including cancer and heart disease combined. It can even be life threatening. For all, arthritis means living with pain and stiffness. That's the bad news.

The good news is that there is an alternative approach. Arthritis *can* be prevented and the underlying causes *can* be eliminated. If you stop or reverse the progression of this disease early enough you can hope for a complete recovery. If your arthritis has already resulted in considerable damage to joints you may, at best, be able to halt the progression of the disease and reduce the pain with little or no recourse to drugs. Either way, to find the best approach to treating your arthritis you need to identify the likely factors that contributed to it developing in the first place, which is what Part One of this book is all about. But even before that, it helps to understand the nature of the beast.

What is arthritis?

There are two major kinds of arthritis, and many less common arthritis-like conditions. Osteoarthritis, the most common kind, is a progressive, degenerative 'wear and tear' disease. Rheumatoid arthritis is less common and less understood. It affects younger people and seems to be associated with a faulty immune system, perhaps triggered by hereditary factors and infections, as well as diet and lifestyle.

A healthy joint consists of bone with a layer of smooth, less brittle cartilage, separated from the opposite bone by a lubricating synovial fluid kept within the area by surrounding synovial membrane.

BONE consists of a matrix of collagen, a kind of protein, which binds in the minerals calcium, phosphorus and magnesium. Calcium is the greatest single constituent of bone, with 99 per cent of the body's calcium found within bone.

CARTILAGE consists of proteoglycans, a kind of mucopolysaccharide made from protein and carbohydrate. Cartilage is smooth and less brittle than bone, thereby protecting the bone ends and maintaining smooth joint movements.

SYNOVIAL FLUID is a lubricating liquid produced in synovial cells and secreted into the joint space to lubricate the joint.

SYNOVIAL MEMBRANE surrounds the joint space enclosing the synovial fluid.

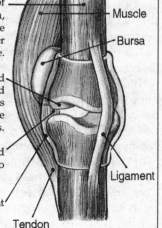

Muscle

Bursa

Ligament

Tendon

Figure 1 A Healthy Joint

•Osteoarthritis

About 80 per cent of people over the age of 50 show *osteoarthritis*-like joint damage, a quarter of which experience pain. By the age of 60 over 90 per cent of people show evidence on X-ray of arthritis-like joint damage. While osteoarthritis occurs later in life, knee problems, often diagnosed as chondromalacia, occur frequently in people less than 40 years of age.

Under the age of 45 osteoarthritis is more common in men; over the age of 45 it's more common in women, probably due to reduced calcium absorption after the menopause. It starts as stiffness, usually of the weight bearing joints such as the knees, hips and back, and then progresses to pain on movement. The joints then become increasingly swollen and inflexible.

Osteoarthritis is marked by a loss of *cartilage* (see Figure 1) which is made from *proteoglycans,* a kind of *mucopolysaccharide* that we will talk about later on in this book. Loss of cartilage leads to excess friction and overuse. This in turn leads to drying out of the cartilage and further loss of cartilage. This loss affects the health of the bone ends as collagen, the protein matrix of bone, starts to break down. This leads to a thickening of bone ends and the formation of *osteophytes* which are large bone spurs, often making the joint appear enlarged. *Synovial fluid* becomes stickier and less able to lubricate. The whole joint area becomes increasingly inflamed, and movement becomes increasingly restricted. Calcium, instead of being incorporated into bone, may get dumped in other tissues of the body, such as muscle, leading to muscle pain and stiffness. Boney protusions, called osteophytes, can form around the joint. In severe osteoarthritis, as the joint becomes immobilised, the bones can fuse together.

Osteoarthritis is usually triggered by either 'wear and tear', for example bad posture plus an insufficient diet to maintain healthy joints, or a trauma such as a strain, obesity, or another disease. The major causes are thought to be improper diet and lifestyle, which, over the years can upset the body's metabolism and ability to keep joints healthy. The progression of osteoarthritis suggests that the body is trying to heal damaged tissue within the joint.

When there is evidence of joint damage, but no pain or inflammation, the condition is called *arthrosis*.

●Rheumatoid arthritis

There are an estimated half a million people in Britain with rheumatoid arthritis. Around 80 per cent of these are women. While the peak age is 30 to 50 many people develop rheumatoid arthritis as young as 25. Unlike osteoarthritis this condition often affects the whole body, and usually both sides of the body, for example both wrists, rather than simply a weight bearing joint. It most often affects fingers, wrists, knees and ankles but can also affect other parts of the body such as heart tissue and muscles.

Rheumatoid arthritis starts with inflammation of the synovial membrane. Consequently the joint becomes inflamed and enlarged. The synovial membrane actual produces chemicals that further

1 A healthy joint consists of strong bones, which are essentially minerals in a collagen (protein) matrix; cartilage on the edge of bone, protected from the opposing bone and cartilage by a sack containing synovial fluid, which effectively lubricates the joint.

2 Cartilage is made from mucopolysaccharides and collagen. Overuse and dietary imbalances can lead to a breakdown of cartilage. Synovial fluid becomes less lubricating. Loss of cartilage also leads to break down of collagen components. Bone ends become uneven and osteophytes (large bone spurs) form. Inflammation restricts movement.

3 Loss of calcium balance can lead to calcium being dumped in soft tissues, causing muscle pain. In rheumatoid arthritis (A) bone ends can become fused together. The goal is to allow the body to rebuild its collagen matrix and restore healthy bones, cartilage and synovial membrane.

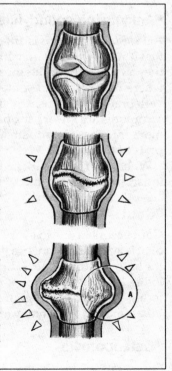

Figure 2 How Arthritis Develops

irritate the joint and start a process of cartilage and, ultimately, bone degeneration. Rheumatoid joints are often warm and the sufferer can have slight fever. They feel tired and generally run down.

The cause is more mysterious but points to immune system problems, either triggered by a viral or bacterial infection, or a genetic weakness. Rheumatoid arthritis often starts and flares up when nutrition is under par, probably because nutrition is vital for immune strength. Most rheumatoid arthritis sufferers develop antibodies which attack normal components of the body, as if the immune system has gone haywire. This is why rheumatoid arthritis is often called an auto-immune disease. It is thought that rheumatoid arthritis is, in part, hereditary.

•Ankylosing spondylitis

Ankylosing spondylitis is different from other arthritic conditions in that it starts with inflammation of the ends of the ligaments where they attach to bone. This most common starts in the sacroiliac joint, where the pelvis and spine meet. As the disease progresses the vertebrae at the base of the spine start to fuse together.The symptoms are lower back pain and stiffness. As the area becomes more inflamed, joint pain and stiffness may also occur in other parts of the body.

When there is evidence of spinal fusion, but no pain or inflammation, the condition is called *spondylosis*.

•Gout

Gout occurs in one in every 200 people. It is caused by a build up of uric acid, a substance in the blood that should be excreted from the body via the kidneys. Excess uric acid can form crystals which lodge in joints and tissue, most commonly the big toe, causing localised pain. When gout is present there is usually increased inflammation which may affect other joints.

•Osteoporosis

Osteoporosis is the gradual loss of bone density. As such it is not specifically a disease of the joints, but of the bones themselves.

However, the health of bones does affect joints, and many underlying mechanisms now thought to contribute to osteoporosis are shared with osteoarthritis.

Osteoporosis is thought to affect over 2 million people in Britain. It occurs twice as commonly in women, and is most prevalent in women after the menopause. It is usually only identified when a fracture occurs, usually of the hip, and it is therefore considered a hidden epidemic. Forty people die every day as a result of fractures due to osteoporosis. Loss of bone density occurs because calcium is not being properly deposited in bone, or is actively being removed. Many factors are known to upset the calcium balance in bone. These include excess protein consumption, excess tea, coffee or alcohol, blood sugar problems, thyroid or parathyroid hormone imbalances, loss of oestrogen production at the menopause, lack of weight bearing exercise, lack of magnesium, lack of vitamin D or sunlight as well as a lack of dietary calcium. These are covered in more detail in Part Three of this book.

● Polymyalgia

Polymyalgia is an increasingly common problem mainly affecting older women in which muscles, rather than joints, become stiff and painful. The onset is usually rapid and suggests that the problem is triggered in some way, perhaps by a virus, or accumulated stress - 'the last straw that broke the camel's back' - initiating a rheumatoid-like condition. There is usually evidence of inflammation. Polymyalgia can spontaneously vanish. Little is known about this condition.

●Osteomalacia or rickets

Osteomalacia (in adults) and rickets (in children) is a disease caused by a deficiency of vitamin D. This vitamin is needed to use calcium properly. A lack of it leads to weak and pliable bones, resulting in bone deformities such as bow legs or bent fingers and toes. Vitamin D is made in the skin in the presence of sunlight, so both diet and exposure of skin play a part. People with dark skin, who get little direct exposure to sunlight, and eat a vegan diet, without eggs, dairy products, meat or fish, are most at risk.

●Displaced intervertebral disc

Displaced intervertebral disc, wrongly referred to as a 'slipped disc', occurs when two vertebrae in the spine are out of alignment which can put pressure on the spinal nerve that runs through the spinal column. Poor spinal alignment can also lead to rupture of the synovial sac between vertebrae, causing tremendous pain both from inflammation and through nerve compression. Eventually the vertebrae can fuse together.

●Bursitis, tendonitis and tenosynovitis

These three inflammatory conditions do not affect joints as such. *Bursitis* refers to inflammation of fluid filled cushions that separate muscle from bone. The most common sites are in the shoulders, elbows and knees. *Tendonitis* is inflammation of where the tendons attach to bone, and *tenosynovitis* is inflammation of the sheath surrounding the tendon.

Terms such as 'lumbago' (back ache) and 'rheumatism' (systemic joint and muscle ache) usually refer to a condition that can be described more accurately by one of the above.

Understanding Research

In the chapters which follow I will refer to many research trials carried out to test different causes of and approaches to the treatment of arthritis. I have tended to avoid anecdotal reports of arthritis cures, unless to illustrate a proven approach or to highlight a potential area for more research, because it is hard to know to what extent the treatment will work for others. The best studies are 'controlled, double-blind trials' with objective and subjective measures of improvement.

For example, an objectively measured increased flexibility of a joint, and a decrease in the *erythrocyte sedimentation rate* in the blood (ESR) which indicates inflammation, are both strong evidence that something has really happened. If backed up by subjective improvement, in other words the patient feels better, this is even better since that is, after all, what treatment sets out to do. However it is important to know if the disease process is being arrested or if the pain is simply being killed.

Controlled studies involve comparisons between two similar groups of people, one receiving the treatment in question, the other not. Sometimes both groups remain on pain killers, but the 'experimental' group also have vitamins. This answers the question as to whether vitamins and pain killers are more effective than pain killers alone. However the effect could be in the mind if you know you're taking vitamins. Some researchers use patients as their own control by monitoring them without treatment, then administering treatment and recording the difference. However you have to take into account whether the disease would have got worse or better anyway.

For this reason scientists love 'double blind' trials. This means that a group of people are given either, for example, a supplement, or a dummy 'placebo' supplement. Neither the person nor the experimenter knows which until the trial is over and the code is broken. The difference between results in one group and the other cannot, therefore, be caused by a psychological effect or by bias on the part of the experimenter. Double blind trials do, however, pose certain ethical problems.

A few words of caution:
1 Never stop or change medication prescribed by your doctor without his or her knowledge and consent.
2 Do not exceed the doses of vitamins, minerals, or amino acids stated in this book.
3 Preferably carry out these recommendations under the guidance of a nutrition consultant (see page 158 for details).
4 If you have adverse reactions to any nutrients it is best to see either your doctor or a qualified nutrition consultant, and stop taking the supplement you suspect of causing a reaction.

While all the recommendations made in this book are based on proper research, and involve substances with minimal or no known risk of adverse reactions, the author cannot be responsible for the outcome of your choosing to experiment with these recommendations.

Now that you know a little more about the nature of arthritis-like diseases, let's look at the new theories about their cause, and new breakthroughs in their treatment.

Part 1

New Theories, New Breakthroughs

1
Why Arthritis?

When you get ill two questions usually come to mind. The first is 'how do I get better?' and the second is 'why did I get ill in the first place?'. Knowing why you develop a disease doesn't cure the disease, but it is usually the first step towards a solution. In the search for the cause of arthritis many things have been considered, including diet, physical exercise, posture, climate, hormones, infections, genetics, old age and stress. Most of these factors have proven relevant to some arthritis suffers. But what is the cause? I believe the answer is, as for most diseases, that arthritis does not have a single cause. The occurrence of the symptoms of arthritis, or any arthritic type of disease, is the result of an accumulation of factors, of stresses that eventually cause joint, bone and muscle degeneration.

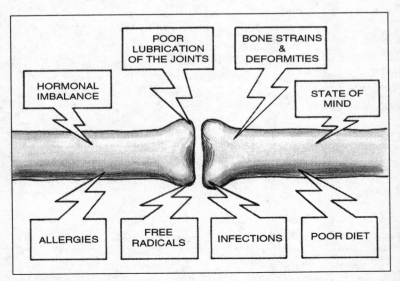

Figure 3 *Factors that Affect the Bones*

The likely factors that lead to the development of this painful condition are:

- **Poor lubrication of the joints**. In between joints there is synovial fluid. Good nutrition is needed to make sure the synovial fluid stays fluid and able to lubricate. Cartilage and synovial fluid contain mucopolysaccharides which can be provided by certain foods.

- **Hormonal imbalance**. Hormones control calcium balance in the body. If calcium balance is out of control bones and joints can become porous and subject to wear and tear, and calcium can be deposited in the wrong place resulting in arthritic 'spurs'. The fault is not so much calcium intake, but the loss of calcium balance in the body. A lack of exercise, excess tea, coffee, alcohol or chocolate, exposure to toxic metals like lead, excessive stress or underlying blood sugar or thyroid imbalances all upset calcium control. While calcium control can be worse after the menopause probably due to the loss of *oestrogen*, too much oestrogen also makes arthritis worse. It's all a question of balance. Another hormone, insulin, stimulates the synthesis of mucopolysaccharides, from which cartilage is made [1]. People with underactive *thyroid glands* are more likely to suffer from arthritis.

- **Allergies and sensitivities**. Almost all rheumatoid arthritics and many osteoarthritics have food and chemical allergies or sensitivities that make their symptoms flare up. The most common food allergies are to wheat and dairy produce. Chemical and environmental sensitivities can include gas and exhaust fumes. These are well worth avoiding strictly for one month to see whether they contribute to the problem.

- **Free radicals.** In all inflamed joints, a battle is taking place, with the body trying to deal with the damage. One of the key weapons of war in the body are free oxidising radicals. These are like the body's own nuclear waste, made from oxygen reacting with glucose, the end result of breathing and eating. The reaction releases energy that allows our cells to work, but it also creates these dangerous oxygen by-products which can destroy cells and damage body tissue. A certain amount of free oxidising radicals, or free radicals for short, are made through normal body processes. Eating a lot of fried food, or smoking cigarettes will increase free radicals in the body. The body protects itself from free radicals with an army of anti-oxidant nutrients, like vitamins A,C and E, and anti-oxidant enzymes which contain the minerals zinc and selenium. In fact, the body will even generate free radicals to destroy abnormal cells or invaders such as a virus. If the immune system isn't working properly, as in rheumatoid arthritis, it will produce too many free radicals which can damage tissue around the joint. A low intake of anti-oxidant nutrients can make arthritis worse.

- **Infections**. Any infection, be it viral or bacterial, weakens the immune system which controls inflammation. But some viruses and bacteria particularly affect the joints by lodging in them and recurring when immune defences are low. Often the immune system can do harm to surrounding tissue in an attempt to fight an infection, like an army which obliterates its own country in trying to get rid of an invader. Building up your immune defences through optimum nutrition is the natural solution.

- **Bone strain and deformities**. Any damage or strain, so often caused by faulty posture, increases the risk of developing arthritis. A yearly check up with an osteopath or chiropractor, plus regular exercise that helps to increase joint suppleness and strength is the best prevention. Once arthritis has set in, special exercises help to reduce pain and stiffness.

- **State of mind**. Research at the Arthritis and Rheumatism Foundation and at the University of Southern California Medical School has shown a link between arthritis and emotional stress. "Hidden anger, fear or worry often accompanies the beginning of arthritis" says Dr Austin from the University of Southern California.

- **Poor diet.** Most arthritics show a history of poor diet which paves the way for many of the above risk factors. Too much refined sugar, too many stimulants, too much fat and too much protein are all strongly associated with arthritic problems. A lack of any of a large number of vital vitamins, minerals and essential fatty acids could, in itself, precipitate joint problems.

According to Dr Robert Bingham, a specialist in the treatment of arthritis "No person who is in good nutritional health develops rheumatoid or osteoarthritis."

By taking all these factors into account and eliminating possible risks, improving lifestyle, and following an optimal diet and supplement programme based on your individual needs, great results can be achieved with arthritis. Pain and inflammation can be reduced, mobility can be increased, and, although less easy to achieve, there is evidence that damaged joints can heal. Each of these factors are discussed in more detail later on in this book.

2
The Conventional Approach

Most conventional treatments for arthritis treat the symptoms, not the cause. The three most common drugs used for arthritic conditions are aspirin, cortisone and NSAID drugs (*Non-Steroidal Anti-Inflammatory Drugs*).

Aspirin - help or hindrance?

The first drug that is often employed is aspirin. It can be quite effective in relieving both pain and inflammation. However, since the amount often needed to make a difference is relatively high (2 to 4 grams a day) toxic side-effects do occur. The early warning signs of toxicity include *tinnitus* (ringing in the ears) and gastric irritation. Aspirin is a completely unnatural substance for the human body. As one doctor said "has anyone ever suffered from a deficiency of aspirin?". The body reacts to it as an irritant. In 1980 the sixth World Nutrition Congress reported that even a single aspirin can cause intestinal bleeding for one week. Just imagine what high doses on a daily basis over many years are likely to do. One side-effect that is rarely mentioned is aspirin's inhibition of synthesis of the collagen matrix that makes up bone, and acceleration of the destruction of cartilage, which has been shown in experimental studies [2]. Aspirin also lowers blood vitamin C levels which are so vital for the formation of collagen. In the short-term the use of aspirin may relieve the symptoms, but in the long term, it is more likely to progress the disease.

The Cortisone Dilemma

Cortisone, or steroid based drugs (such as prednisone, prednisolone, betamethasone etc) are probably the most common prescription for arthritic conditions. Since cortisone's discovery, more than 40 years ago, 101 uses have been found for this potent drug, including the treatment of arthritis. Cortisone is a derivative of a hormone produced naturally by the body, in the adrenal cortex which sits on top of each kidney. As long ago as 1948 Dr Hench, who later won a Nobel prize, reported miraculous results with crippled arthritis suffers. Now, in America 29 million prescriptions are written out each year and, not surprisingly, cortisone is big business. But the belief that cortisone was the cure for arthritis was not long lasting. In one early case, a 10-year-old girl who made an amazing recovery from severe arthritis when given cortisone, quickly developed diabetes. When the cortisone was stopped the diabetes went away but the arthritis returned with a vengeance.

Exactly how cortisone works is still not completely understood. What is known is that it reduces inflammation by inhibiting the production of histamine. It also suppresses the immune system, which could be good if your immune system is destroying healthy cells, as in an auto-immune disease like rheumatoid arthritis. It also interferes with the availability to cells of *arachidonic acid*, a fatty acid that encourages the formation of short-lived substances called *leukotrienes* and prostaglandins (type 2), which encourage inflammation.

The trouble is that, once you start taking it, the adrenal glands stop producing it. Given in small amounts cortisone seems manageable, but in large amounts, particularly over long periods of time, the side effects can be disastrous and even deadly. "The sad truth is that, like aspirin, cortisone does not cure anything; it merely suppresses the symptoms of the disease." says Dr Barnett Zumoff of Beth Israel Medical Center in New York City and formerly of the Steroid Research Laboratory at New York's Montefiore Hospital [3]. Withdrawal from high doses of cortisone must be very gradual to allow the adrenal glands to recover production of their own cortisone. Even so, a full recovery is often not possible, leaving previous cortisone users unable to produce enough to respond to stressful situations such as an accident or operation. Severe adrenal insufficiency can be fatal.

Some of the other consequences of long-term cortisone use may not be fatal, but they can be extremely unpleasant. They include obesity, a rounded moon face, a heightened susceptibility to infection, slow wound healing, muscle wasting and congestive heart failure. "Using it," says Dr Zumoff "is like trying to repair a computer with a monkey wrench." While cortisone has undoubtedly saved many lives, its long-term high dose use is unlikely to cure arthritis, and may even speed up the disease, with added undesirable side effects.

NSAIDs - Are They Any Better?

Due to the dangers associated with the use of steroid drugs like cortisone, many varieties of non-steroidal anti-inflammatory drugs have been developed as an alternative. These include ibuprofen (Motrin), fenoprofen (Fenopron), flurbiprofen (Froben), ketoprofen (Alrheumat, Orudis and Oruvail) naproxen (Naprosyn), tolmetin (Tolectin), sulindac (Clinoril), azapropazone (Rheumox), indomethacin (Indocid), phenylbutazone (Butazolidine), mefenamic acid (Ponstan), diclofenac (Voltarol), fenbufen (Lederfen), piroxicam (Feldene), tiaprofenic acid (Surgam), tolmetin (Tolectin). In Britain alone 22 million prescriptions are written for these drugs each year. NSAIDs seem to work mainly by blocking the effect of the inflammatory prostaglandins (type 2), which are hormone-like substances in the body derived from essential fatty acids from the diet.

NSAIDs are responsible for many toxic reactions and often cause undesirable side-effects. These include headaches, dizziness and digestive complaints such as nausea, vomiting, diarrhoea and intestinal bleeding, and should therefore only be recommended for short periods of time, if at all [4]. The use of NSAIDs has also been associated with increased gut permeability [5] and ulcers in the small intestine which can have serious complications. It has been suggested that a large proportion of hitherto unexplained ulcers in the small intestine may be due to these drugs [6]. At least nine NSAID drugs have been withdrawn, including Opren. Approximately one quarter of all adverse drug reactions reported are for NSAIDs.

Although NSAIDs are sometimes better tolerated and more effective than aspirin they too inhibit the synthesis of collagen and accelerate the destruction of cartilage, thus speeding up the progression of arthritis [7]. NSAIDs should be reduced slowly as an abrupt end to medication often makes symptoms flare up.

3

Reducing Pain & Inflammation without Drugs

Both NSAIDs and steroid drugs may reduce inflammation by affecting *prostaglandins*. Prostaglandins are short-lived, hormone-like substances in the body, derived from essential fats found in the diet. While one group of prostaglandins (prostaglandin type 2) encourage inflammation, another group of prostaglandins, known as PGE1 (prostaglandin type 1) have been shown to reduce inflammation in animals in a variety of studies [8].

PGEI is derived from linoleic acid, found in seeds and their oils. Sesame, sunflower and safflower oil are particularly rich sources of these essential fatty acids. In turn, the body converts linoleic acid into gamma-linolenic acid (GLA), and then on to *di-homo gamma-linolenic acid* (DGLA), which then goes to form prostaglandins, as shown in Figure 4. The conversion step from linoleic acid to gamma linolenic acid is not so efficient in some people, depending on an enzyme (delta-six-desaturase) which is itself dependent on an adequate supply of vitamin B6, biotin, zinc and magnesium. Another converting enzyme (delta-5-desaturase) depends on vitamin C and B3 (niacin). The ability to convert the essential fats in seeds into anti-inflammatory prostaglandins is also hampered in older people, by a diet high in saturated fat, by alcohol, smoking and stress.

For these reasons GLA, the pre-converted essential fat, which is rich in evening primrose oil and borage oil, has been used effectively as an anti-inflammatory nutrient. GLA has been shown to be effective in the treatment of arthritis [9], arthritis associated with a bacterial infection [10], and inflammation caused by high uric acid levels, the cause of gout [11].

Evening primrose oil has proven at least as effective as NSAIDs

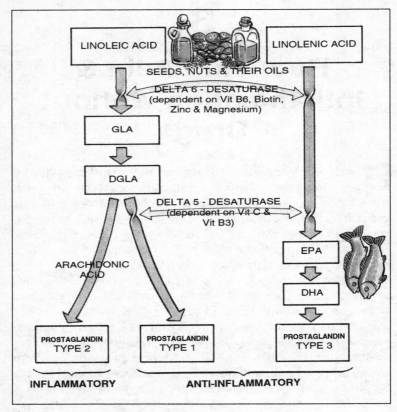

Figure 4 From Essential Fatty Acids to Prostaglandins

in reducing inflammation and the symptoms of rheumatoid arthritis in two trials to date. The first, unwisely stopped NSAID medication abruptly, substituting evening primrose oil for a period of twelve weeks [12]. While there was no improvement in the arthritis there was a reduction in inflammation and only 2 out of the 17 patients deteriorated, whereas most of them would have been expected to deteriorate coming off NSAID medication. This study suggests that sources of GLA, such as evening primrose oil, may be at least as effective as anti-inflammatory drugs without the same risk of side-effects.

In a much longer trial comparing the effects of essential fatty acids with NSAIDs the results were definitely positive 13. Arthritic patients, stable on NSAIDs, were assigned to one of three groups. One received 100% evening primrose oil, the other 80% evening primrose oil and 20% fish oil, and the third a placebo (dummy pill). After three months patients were encouraged to reduce or stop altogether their NSAID medication over the next nine months. At the end of this time, everyone was put on placebos. About 90 per cent of those taking essential fatty acids reported improvement and were able to stop, or at least considerably reduce the NSAIDs, compared to 30 per cent in the placebo group. Almost all who had improved on essential fatty acids regressed when placed on the placebo.

As a natural anti-inflammatory nutrient GLA, found in evening primrose oil and borage, is likely to be at least as effective as NSAIDs in the long-run, without side-effects or the risk of speeding up the progression of the disease. Whether essential fatty acid supplementation halts or slows down the progression of arthritis is not yet known, however it should reduce inflammation and consequently, the pain.

The amount of GLA required to have this effect is quite high, and consequently, quite expensive unless given on prescription. I recommend 300mg of GLA per day, reducing to 150mg after three months if inflammation reduces and symptoms stay stable. Only 9 to 10 per cent of the oil in evening primrose oil is from GLA so that means at least 3,000mg of evening primrose oil, or six 500mg capsules per day. Borage oil contains a higher proportion of GLA and you can get capsules which provide 150mg of GLA. Two of these each day would reach the suggested intake for the first three months.

Supplementing GLA has been shown to be more effective when the co-factor vitamins and minerals (vitamin B6, zinc, B3 and vitamin C) are also supplied 14.

Oiling the Joints

Another kind of essential fatty acid is found in oily fish, particularly herring, mackerel, salmon and shark. This is derived from an essential oil called linolenic acid, which is found in nuts and seeds.

The richest source is linseed, sometimes called flax seed, and its oil. Linolenic acid is also found in plankton, which the small fish eat. When larger fish eat small fish they start to concentrate and convert linolenic acid into two complex fatty acids that can again be used by the body to produce prostaglandins. These are EPA (eicosapentaenoic acid) and DHA (docosahexaenoic acid). Smaller amounts of these fatty acids are also found in other fish oils such as cod liver oil.

Studies have also confirmed that supplementing these fish oils helps reduce the symptoms of arthritis. In one study 17 patients were given 1.8g of EPA a day. After twelve weeks they had significantly less stiffness and tenderness of joints. The improvement didn't last once the patients stopped taking the EPA supplements [15]. These positive results were confirmed in another study which gave rheumatoid arthritis patients on NSAID medication 10 fish oil capsules daily. After six weeks there was a significant reduction in the number of painful joints in those taking fish oil compared to those simply on NSAIDs. When the NSAID medication was withdrawn this improvement vanished, however there was no deterioration in symptoms beyond that level experienced when on NSAIDs, which would have been expected [16]. A further trial on 16 rheumatoid arthritic patients also demonstrated positive results for fish oils over 12 weeks [17].

In a further study Dr Kremer and his colleagues showed that the dose of fish oil, and the length of time taken both have an important effect on the relief experienced [18]. They gave 49 patients with active rheumatoid arthritis either low dose fish oil (providing 27mg/kg of EHA and 18mg/kg of DHA), high dose fish oil (providing 54mg/kg EPA and 36mg/kg DHA) or olive oil, under double-blind conditions. They monitored changes over 24 weeks. Improvements in tender joints were most marked in the high dose fish oil group after 24 weeks, while joint swelling decreased significantly after only 12 weeks. Results were best in the high fish oil group. Of the 45 different clinical measures taken to monitor change, 21 improved in the high dose group, 8 in the low dose group and 5 in the olive oil group.

The benefits of fish oil was confirmed last year by a study undertaken in three Danish hospitals [19]. Fifty one patients with rheumatoid arthritis were given either six fish oil capsules (giving 3.6g of fish oil equivalent to 1,200mg of EPA) or capsules containing fat with the composition of the normal Danish diet. Although the dosage of EPA was somewhat lower than earlier trials the results showed a clear improvement in joint tenderness and morning stiffness.

This strongly suggests that large enough amounts of fish oil, probably due to its EPA and DHA content, is anti-inflammatory and may be as effective as NSAID medication in some cases, without the side-effects. It is likely that the anecdotal reports of cod liver oil helping arthritis stem from the fact that cod liver oil contains EPA and DHA. However, cod itself has a much lower EPA content than mackerel, herring and salmon.

One word of caution: both fish oil and aspirin thin the blood. The combined use of large amounts of both could lead to a potentially harmful inability of blood to clot, hence long bleeding times on injury. Therefore it may be prudent not to combine on-going aspirin and high dose fish oil [20].

Natural Pain Control

Pain is the body's way of alerting us to a problem. While different people have differing abilities to tolerate pain it is unwise to ignore pain and exercise a joint to the point where inflammation is increased. This can only make your arthritis worse. Overuse of some pain killing drugs may not only speed up the progression of arthritis but also unwisely allow a joint to be overused. It is therefore best to use pain killers as little as possible, without causing yourself unnecessary suffering.

Your body is made out of mainly water (65 per cent) and protein (25 per cent). All the different kinds of protein in the body are made out of combinations of 23 different kinds of amino acids, much in the same way that millions of words are made out the 26 letters of the alphabet. Some of these amino acids have important parts to play in the chemistry of the brain. One amino acid, called *phenylalanine*, may allow the body's natural pain killers to act for longer. The body has the ability to produce immensely powerful pain inhibitors, known as opiod peptides, such as enkephalins. These substances are 10 to 1000 times more potent than morphine but, unfortunately, their action is short lived. Dl-phenylalanine has been shown to extend their life span by inhibiting the enzymes that break them down. Phenylalanine comes in two forms, d-phenylalanine (DPA), or dl-phenylalanine, *(DLPA)*. DPA or DLPA can be bought as a supplement in health food shops and has proven effective in relieving chronic pain, even when standard medication has given limited or no relief.

In one study 43 patients, mainly with osteoarthritis, were supplemented with DPA 250mg three to four times daily for four to five weeks. Significant pain reduction was reported among osteoarthritis sufferers, especially during the last two weeks [21]. In another study in which 21 chronic pain patients were given either placebo pills or DPA, 7 patients on DPA experienced 50% pain relief, which was not maintained when they were switched onto a placebo. The remaining 13 patients had no significant relief of pain from DPA [22]. These studies followed up an earlier study which showed good to total relief of pain in a group of ten patients including those with osteoarthritis, rheumatoid arthritis and low back pain after only 3 days on DPA [23].

Not all studies have reported benefit from the use of DPA or DLPA [24]. The results of these studies suggest that the effects are accumulative and may only appear after two weeks of supplementation in some cases. Some people seem to obtain good pain relief from DPA or DLPA, while others don't. One 47 year-old woman, who had had rheumatoid arthritis for 18 years with severe swelling of the hands to the point where you couldn't see her knuckles, tried DLPA. Within seven days the pain and swelling reduced so dramatically that her knuckles became visible and her joints became flexible [25].

The recommended dose is 250mg of DPA (or 750mg of DLPA) 3 times a day for three weeks. If this dose is ineffective you may wish to try a higher dose, however this should not be done without the supervision of your doctor or a qualified nutrition consultant, as high doses of amino acids can also have side-effects. Side-effects associated with excessive DPA or DLPA include increased anxiety, high blood pressure or headaches. Since amino acids in food compete with each other for absorption into the body, DPA or DLPA are best taken 15 to 30 minutes before a meal on an empty stomach, or with juice.

4

The Cartilage Connection

The fact that some individuals develop arthritis at an early age, that it is more common in women and can strike whole families, strongly suggests that something other than 'wear and tear' is involved. It is reasonable to consider that there may be differences between people in their health or ability to regenerate healthy cartilage since it is the degeneration of cartilage that seems to herald the beginning of osteoarthritis, the common form of this ailment. Cartilage of osteoarthritic sufferers does appear to be different in composition from that of non-sufferers [26].

What is Cartilage?

Cartilage is the 'gristle' in meat. In our bodies the Adam's apple, tip of our nose, bone ends, and shock absorbers between spinal vertebrae are all made of cartilage. It is a tough, elastic and translucent material. The kind of cartilage at bone ends is called fibrocartilage and is the strongest of all.

In foetal development cartilage forms the framework for the body, which then becomes calcified to produce bones. The bones of children are more pliable because they contain more cartilage and less calcium. At the tops of bones are regions called 'growth plates', where the cartilage develops, allowing bones to grow. Once calcification of cartilage has occurred this process cannot be reversed.

Cells that produce cartilage are called *chondrocytes* which produce cartilaginous fibres. Cartilage is made of a complex of protein, polysaccharides and collagen, a kind of intercellular glue. This complex is what is thought to give cartilage its special properties. Much research has focused on ways of improving the body's ability to make healthy cartilage and heal joints. To this effect extracts from shark cartilage and green lipped mussels have entered the repertoire of arthritis remedies. As bizarre as this sounds there is good reason. The green lipped muscle contains

31

high levels of protein, vitamins and minerals, and a special ingredient called 'mucopolysaccharides' which is a natural joint lubricant and component of all cartilage. Shark cartilage, a recent addition to health food shop shelves, may have a similar effect.

The theory, in accord with the basic principle of 'optimum nutrition' is that if you provide your body cells with the materials they need to do their job properly, they will. If arthritics lack the necessary components to make healthy cartilage, why not provide it? It is certainly far less invasive than giving drugs that suppress the symptoms but do nothing to stop the disease. Unlike other body tissue cartilage has no blood or nerve supply. Cartilage relies on nutrients within the fluid of the body which is moved around joint spaces by compression and relaxation. Thus exercise is another way to improve nutrient transport to cartilage. During the day the cartilaginous discs between spinal verterbrae compresses. At night, when we lie down, these discs expand sucking in nutrients from surrounding body fluids.

Relief from the Ocean?

Proper controlled studies have shown benefit for both rheumatoid arthritis and osteoarthritis sufferers from supplementing green lipped mussel extract. While most people make enough mucopolysaccharides there is evidence that arthritics don't. Supplementing may help.

In one study of 55 patients given green lipped mussel extract for 6 months to 4.5 years, 67 per cent benefited [27]. In a double-blind study 28 patients receiving NSAID medication were given either green lipped mussel extract (350mg three times a day) or a placebo, for six months. Those taking the green lipped mussel extract did significantly better than those taking the placebos [28].

A higher proportion of rheumatoid arthritis sufferers receive benefit from green lipped mussel extract. This supports other research which suggests that mucopolysaccharides, as well as being components of healthy cartilage, have a significant anti-inflammatory effect.

The recommended dose of green lipped mussel extract is 1,000mg a day for 25 days then 250mg a day. Some people experience a flare up of symptoms within the first two weeks, before their condition improves. Obviously, this is not suitable for people with a known seafood allergy.

Sharks Don't get Arthritis

Another rich source of mucopolysaccharides is cartilage itself. Two sources of cartilage extract have been investigated in relation to arthritis. One from calves, the other from sharks.

In one study 28 patients with severe osteoarthritis were given injections of Catrix (cartilage extract) over a period of 3 to 8 weeks. 19 were classified as 'excellent results', 6 'good', 2 received some benefit and 1 had no discernible change. In a study of 9 rheumatoid arthritis patients 3 were reported as having an excellent response, and 6 a good response [29].

Sharks, unlike most mammals, contain no bones. Their skeleton is completely composed of cartilage. About 7 per cent of a shark's weight is cartilage compared to 1 per cent for mammals. Numerous research trials have been conducted on shark cartilage in relation to cancer [30]. Shark cartilage has been shown to stop cancer cells from developing the blood supply they need to survive and grow. Preventing this process, known as anti-angiogenesis, may also have significance for arthritis since *angiogenesis*, or vascularisation, seems to occur in the joints of rheumatoid arthritics, leading to more rapid breakdown of cartilage [31]. So rich mucopolysaccharide sources may prevent inflammation, and breakdown of cartilage and encourage the formation of healthy, new cartilage.

Dr Serge Orloff, European secretary for the International Association of Rheumatologists, decided to experiment with shark cartilage on his arthritic patients [32]. He started with 9 grams a day for four weeks, and then halved the dose for a further four weeks. The results were good, especially in one 49 year-old woman with joint disease and low back pain attributable to disc degeneration. Her pain rating decreased by 50% after two weeks and a further 50% after six weeks, by which time she had greatly increased mobility and less pain. According to Dr Lane, in his book Sharks Don't Get Cancer, eastern European studies have shown great improvement with cartilage preparations given over many years, including an 85% decrease in pain, compared to a control group given NSAID medication or placebos who only had a 5% decrease in pain.

These beneficial reports of shark cartilage have been confirmed by Dr Orcasita, assistant clinical professor at the University of Miami School of Medicine 33, and by Dr Alpizar in Costa Rica who treated 10 bedridden patients with osteoarthritis 34. Within three weeks 8 were able to walk.

Shark cartilage is also good for dogs, according to Dr Rauis, a vet from Brussels 35. He treated 10 dogs with osteoarthritis and found significant decrease in joint swelling and increased mobility. However, to date, no properly controlled double-blind trial on shark cartilage has been completed, which is hardly surprising since the discovery of its potential therapeutic effect is very recent. Until such trials are carried out the relative effectiveness of shark cartilage cannot be judged, however it may well be worth experimenting with. The only source of shark cartilage I have been able to find in Britain is Cartilade, made by the Solgar vitamin company (see The Directory on page 154).

Building Blocks for Healthy Joints

Amino acids are the building blocks of protein. Two in particular, methionine and cystine, may have an important role to play in restoring joint health. Methionine and its 'cousin' S adenosyl methionine (SAM), are important for synthesising proteoglycans and glycoaminoglycans, which are kinds of mucopolysaccharides, essential components of cartilage 36. A double blind trial involving 150 patients has shown SAM to be better than NSAIDs for the treatment of osteoarthritis 37. In another study SAM significantly reduced pain and increased hip and knee flexibility in osteoarthritis sufferers 38.

The Vitamin C Connection

Vitamin C is vital for healthy joints. Both bone and cartilage formation depend on collagen as a building material which is only synthesised in the presence of vitamin C. So a lack of vitamin C could quite possibly cause cartilage and bone abnormalities. The optimal intake of vitamin C is highly debatable. At the low end of the scale are government set Recommended Daily Amounts (RDAs), usually around 45 to 60mg per day. On the other hand, there is open recognition that the optimal levels needed to protect against cancer and heart disease may be considerably above 1,000mg a day. Why the difference?

Vitamin C isn't a vitamin at all. It isn't a necessary component of diet, at least for all mammals with the exception of guinea pigs, fruit eating bats, the bulbul bird and primates, which includes us. Scientists believe that a negative mutation may have occurred 25 million years ago to cause us to lose the ability to make vitamin C.

Mutations can and frequently do occur in nature. Only those that put a species at advantage at the time tend to become dominant. Unfortunately, reversing such mutations is highly unlikely to occur. Unlike other vitamins, vitamin C is required in large amounts which could only be supplied by a tropical diet high in fruit and other vegetation. If sufficient vitamin C could be obtained from such a diet the quantity of glucose normally used to make vitamin C could be used for energy production. This could conceivably have put primates at an advantage over other animals.

This advantage may have come at a price, especially when the climate and diet changed. Only non-vitamin C producing animals are susceptible to certain kinds of diseases, particularly immune based disease 39. Could humanity's history of disease - endemic infections, plagues and more recently cancer, heart disease and rheumatoid arthritis - be the result of our inability to produce vitamin C and our inability to obtain optimal amounts from the food we eat?

The fact that almost all species continue to make vitamin C suggests that the amount generally available from diet is not enough, except possibly in a tropical environment. The daily amount produced by other animals (adjusted for comparison to man) is between 3,000mg and 15,000mg, with an average of 5,400mg 40.

What about us? While a mere 60mg a day can prevent scurvy, a survey of doctors found that those who were healthiest consumed at least 250mg of vitamin C per day. A person's vitamin C status is a good predictor of their mortality risk. High vitamin C levels indicate a low risk for cardiovascular disease and certain types of cancer. Life expectancy of cancer patients has been doubled on 10,000mg (10 g) a day. Optimal intakes to reduce risk of such conditions may be at least 500mg a day.

But aren't you simply making expensive urine when you take large amounts of supplements? Dr Michael Colgan investigated how much vitamin C we use by giving increasing daily doses and measuring excretion [41]. "Only a quarter of our subjects reached their vitamin C maximum at 1,500mg a day. More than half required over 2,500mg a day to reach a level where their bodies could use no more. Four subjects did not reach their maximum at 5,000mg."

Vitamin C is not only required for the synthesis of collagen, our intercellular glue that keeps skin, lungs, arteries, the digestive tract and all organs intact. It is a potent anti-oxidant protecting against free radicals, pollution, carcinogens, heavy metals, and other toxins. It is vital for a healthy immune system and is strongly anti-viral and mildly anti-bacterial, and anti-inflammatory. A recent study showed, in the test tube, that vitamin C can even inactivate the HIV virus [42]. Energy cannot be made in any cell, brain or muscle without adequate vitamin C. It is also essential for the body's production of stress hormone synthesis, including natural cortisone.

The optimum intake is likely to be in the region of 1,000mg (1 g) to 10,000mg (10 g) per day. If you suffer from chronic arthritis, particularly rheumatoid arthritis, the ideal level may be in the higher range. If you drink excessive amounts of alcohol, live in a polluted city, have a stressful lifestyle, take drugs including aspirin, or smoke, your optimal intake will be raised. An intake of around 50mg per cigarette probably affords maximum protection.

Albert Szent Gyorgi, who isolated vitamin C in 1928, took 1 gram daily. Dr Michael Colgan takes 5 grams daily. Dr Linus Pauling takes 10 grams daily. I take up to 5 grams daily on top of a vitamin C rich diet. For anyone suffering with arthritis 3 to 5 grams a day would be a sensible daily intake to assist healthy collagen formation of bone and cartilage.

5

Skeletons in the Cupboard

The ability to keep your bones strong, a prerequisite to preventing arthritis and osteoporosis, depends to a large extent on the balance of calcium, magnesium and phosphorus, all of which are incorporated into bone. Of these, calcium status is the most important. More and more evidence is accumulating to show that dietary calcium intake is only one of a number of factors that influence the proper use of calcium in the body[43]. Figure 5 gives a list of factors associated with misuse of calcium in the body.

Take a look at your own diet and lifestyle over the last twenty years. Which of these may have contributed to the state of your bones and joints? Since most of these factors are the direct consequence of diet and lifestyle, which do you think is more likely to help: leaving your diet and lifestyle as it is and taking drugs; or changing your diet and lifestyle for the better? One thing

Factors That Negatively Affect Calcium Balance

Lack of minerals - calcium, magnesium, boron
Lack of vitamins - vitamin D, C and B vitamins
Lack of thyroid and parathyroid hormones
Lack of oestrogen - after the menopause
Lack of exercise
Lack of sunlight

Excess of protein - resulting in high levels of acidity
Excess of refined carbohydrates - resulting in blood sugar problems
Excess of stress
Excess of alcohol - particularly red wine
Excess of stimulants - coffee, tea, cigarettes, chocolate
Excess of toxic elements - lead, cadmium, aluminium, fluorine

Figure 5

is certain. There's a lot more to healthy bones than getting enough calcium. While most of these factors are discussed in depth later on in this book two factors are worth considering here. The first is the danger of too much protein, and the second, the extent to which hormone deficiencies contribute to arthritis and osteoporosis and whether hormone replacement therapy is really advisable.

Protein and Osteoporosis

Osteoporosis is endemic in the Western world, particularly among post-menopausal women. The reason, it is thought, is that the hormone oestrogen, which ceases to be produced at the menopause, assists the absorption of dietary calcium. Consequently, numerous trials have tested the effects of giving oral oestrogen, or calcium, or both. Neither have succeeded in completely 'curing' the problem, although both have an effect. This suggests another cause, obvious when you know that many women from different cultures throughout the world have no increased incidence of osteoporosis after the menopause. Many cultural groups have no osteoporosis at all. The Bantus, in Africa, for example have an average calcium intake of 400mg, well below the recommended intake for post-menopausal women, and virtually no osteoporosis. In contrast, Eskimos, who consume vast amounts of calcium, have an exceptionally high incidence of osteoporosis. Why the difference? What have countries with a high incidence of osteoporosis got in common? The answer may be too much dietary protein [44].

Protein rich foods are acid forming. The body cannot tolerate substantial changes in the acid pH of blood and neutralises or 'buffers' this effect through two main alkaline agents - sodium and calcium. When body reserves of sodium are used up calcium is taken from the bone. Therefore the more protein you eat the more calcium you need. The difference between the Bantus and the Eskimos is their protein consumption.

The fact that high protein diets lead to calcium deficiency is nothing new. But what research is beginning to show is that if you eat a high protein diet no amount of calcium corrects the imbalance. In one study published in the American Journal of Clinical Nutrition [45] subjects were given a moderately high protein diet (12g nitrogen) and a very high protein diet (36g nitrogen) plus

1,400mg of calcium. The overall loss of calcium was 37mg per day on the 12g nitrogen diet and 137mg per day on the 36g nitrogen diet. The authors concluded that "high calcium diets are unlikely to prevent probable bone loss induced by high protein diets." In another study a protein intake of 95 grams a day (bacon and eggs for breakfast supplies 55 grams), resulted in an average calcium loss of 58mg per day, which means a loss of 2% of total skeletal calcium per year, or 20% each decade [46]. The negative effects of too much protein has been clearly demonstrated in patients with osteoporosis [47]. Some medical scientists now believe that a life-long consumption of a high protein, acid-forming diet may be a primary cause of osteoporosis [48].

Is Arthritis a Hormone Deficiency Disease?

The endocrine system forms a network of glands that secrete hormones. The hormones control many of the body processes that happen inside us. Hormones can be protein-like, such as insulin, or fat-like, such as *cortisol*. Fat based hormones are called steroid hormones. Most hormones are themselves controlled by means of feedback. An example of this feedback mechanism is seen by examining the pituitary.

Called the master gland because of its overall control, the pituitary governs the functioning of the thyroid gland, the adrenal glands, and the sex glands. The thyroid gland, in turn, controls our rate of metabolism and, together with the *parathyroid glands*, the balance and utilisation of calcium; the adrenal glands control our ability to deal with stress, and, together with the pancreas, the balance and

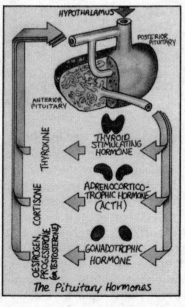

Figure 6 *The endocrine glands and hormones*

39

utilisation of glucose (sugar); while the sex glands control the production of sex hormones, including oestrogen which affects calcium levels. The adrenal glands also produce a small amount of sex hormones.

There is one golden rule of any body organ or system: if you continually over-use or overstress any organ or system it will eventually underfunction. If the entire endocrine system is overstressed this would lead to slow metabolism, calcium imbalance, blood sugar imbalance, inability to cope with stress, sex hormone imbalances and (in women) premature menopause with exaggerated symptoms. After noticing that many of my arthritic patients had a history of prolonged stress, over-use of stimulants, over-consumption of refined carbohydrates, and deficiency of the many essential vitamins and minerals needed for the endocrine system to work, I wondered whether arthritis couldn't be caused, at least in part, by hormone imbalances caused by overstressing the endocrine system as a whole. Rather than treating the effect, in other words giving hormones like cortisone, thyroxine, calcitriol and oestrogen, I experimented with treating the possible cause by encouraging my patients to change their diet and lifestyle and give their endocrine system support through supplements of vitamins and minerals. This approach has proven most effective, and although as yet unproven in clinical trials, research is beginning to confirm that this hypothesis makes sense[49].

Is Oestrogen Really the Answer for Osteoporosis?

The current conventional treatment of osteoporosis is hormone replacement therapy employing oestrogen. There is little doubt that this does increase bone density and reduce the incidence of fracture. However, oestrogen therapy can also increase the risk of hypertension, gall bladder disease, blood clots and, most importantly, uterine or endometrial cancer. To reduce this possibility oestrogen is sometimes supplemented with progesterone, a combination that can cause vaginal bleeding [50]. Stopping oestrogen therapy rapidly returns bone mass to its previous osteoporotic level[51]. Therefore, oestrogen therapy is only really effective as a long-term treatment, which means a long-term risk of potential side effects.

Although not so striking in effect, ensuring adequate intake of calcium, vitamin D and other nutrients, especially magnesium, does increase bone density. Vitamin D is converted into a hormone, calcitriol, that improves calcium utilisation and retention in the body. Supplementing the hormone itself may be even more effective than taking vitamin D, and, unlike oestrogen, carries no apparent significant side effects 52.

A high calcium intake prior to the menopause does seem to improve bone density 53. However, once osteoporosis has set in, calcium supplementation is only marginally effective in increasing bone density except in people who eat a calcium deficient diet. The recommended intake of calcium for a post-menopausal woman is in the order of 1,000 to 1,500mg per day. More than this is most unlikely to be of any benefit.

In conclusion, the best advice for anyone, whether suffering from arthritis or osteoporosis is to avoid excesses of protein, sugar, alcohol and stimulants and to ensure optimal intakes of vitamins and minerals. Even when these factors are taken care of, only if there is evidence of osteoporosis, hormone replacement therapy may still be recommended. However, much lower levels of hormones will be effective, thereby reducing the associated risks. The combined supplementation of vitamins and minerals, plus hormones, has not only proven more effective in restoring bone density, but is more effective in retaining bone density once hormone replacement therapy is stopped 49. Whether or not the complete approach recommended in this book, including diet, low stimulant intake, exercise and supplements, can replace hormone replacement therapy has yet to be put to the test.

Part 2

Diet & Arthritis

6

The Myth of the Balanced Diet

The greatest lie in health care today is that "as long as you eat a well balanced diet you get all the nutrients you need". This is a lie because no single piece of research in the last decade has managed to show that people who consider themselves to be eating a well-balanced diet are receiving all the Recommended Daily Amounts (RDA) of vitamins and minerals, let alone those levels of nutrients that are consistent with optimum nutrition. When conventional nutritionists are asked what a well-balanced diet is, they define it as a diet that provides all the nutrients you need. Catch 22. According to Dr. Stephen Davies these people are "nutritional flat-earthers" because they "employ a thought process akin to that which was adopted by the original 'flat-earthers', those who maintained that the world was flat, rather than round, despite overwhelming evidence to the contrary"[1].

The reality is that the vast majority of us are deficient in a number of essential nutrients, which includes vitamins, minerals, essential fatty acids, and amino acids, the constituents of protein. Deficient, means 'not efficient', in other words that you are not functioning as efficiently as you could because you have an inadequate intake of one or more nutrients. If this comes as a shock consider the following facts.

1 RDA's are not optimum. According to the National Academy of Sciences, who set US RDA's "RDA's are neither minimal requirements nor necessarily optimal levels of intake"[2]. In the UK, the government funds research to define the optimum intake of vitamins C and E to protect against cancer and heart disease, in recognition of the fact that RDA levels are not necessarily optimum[3]. Factors considered to raise one's requirements considerably above RDA levels include alcohol consumption [4], smoking [5], exercise habits, pregnancy, times of stress including puberty and premenstrual phases, pollution, special dietary habits, for example vegetarianism, and chronic illness such as arthritis.

2 RDA's vary from country to country. A five-fold variation from one country to another is not at all uncommon. For example, in Holland the RDA for vitamin A is 333 units, while in Switzerland it's 5,500 units. Why the difference?

3 RDA's don't exist for many essential nutrients. There are 45 known essential nutrients. In Britain RDA's, now known as RNI's (reference nutrient intakes) exist for 20 of these.

4 The majority of people do not achieve RDA levels from their diet. A government survey in 1990 showed that the average person does not get the RDA for iron [6]. An independent survey in 1985 found over 90 per cent of people consumed less than the US RDA for vitamin B6 and folic acid [7]. A government report stated that 10 per cent of the British population consumes less than the 30mg of vitamin C [8], with the UK RNI being 40mg, low in comparison with many other countries which recommend 75mg.

5 Food does not contain what you think it contains. Most of these surveys are based on recording what people eat and looking up what those foods contain in standard text books. But do they take into account that an orange can contain anything from 180mg of vitamin C to nothing [9]? A 100g serving of spinach can contain from 158mg of iron to 0.1mg depending on where it's grown. Wheatgerm can contain from 21ius of vitamin E to 3.2ius. Carrots, that reliable source of vitamin A, can provide a massive 18,500ius down to a mere 70ius. Store an orange for two weeks and its vitamin C content will be halved. Boil a vegetable for 20 minutes and 50 per cent of its B vitamins will be gone [10]. Refine brown flour to make white and 78 per cent of the zinc, chromium and manganese are lost [11]. Today's food is not a reliable source of vitamins and minerals.

Variation in Nutrient Content of Common Foods (per 100g of food)		
Vitamin A	in carrots	70 to 18,500iu
Vitamin B5	in wholewheat flour	0.3 to 3.3mg
Vitamin C	in oranges	0 to 116mg
Vitamin E	in wheatgerm	3.2 to 21iu
Iron	in spinach	0.1 to 158mg
Manganese	in lettuce	0.1 to 16.9mg

Figure 7

6 There is a sliding scale of deficiency. Even if we all ate the RDA levels some people would still show signs of deficiency. For the vast majority these would not be the severe symptoms of scurvy, beriberi or pellagra, but they may well show symptoms such as skin problems, lethargy, poor concentration, frequent infections, allergies and joint aches.

The sad truth is that more suffering is caused by malnutrition, both in the West, and in less developed countries, than by any other cause. According to the US Surgeon General, of the 2.1 million Americans who die each year, 1.5 million, 68 per cent, die from diet related diseases. In Britain three quarters of people die from cardiovascular disease, cancer and the complications of diabetes, all of which are clearly associated with dietary excesses, deficiencies or environmental factors. At the Institute for Optimum Nutrition, where I practise, we give nutritional advice for people with a wide range of problems including digestive disorders, skin problems, cardiovascular disease, cancer, infections, headaches, hormonal problems, diabetes, as well as arthritis. We have an improvement rate of 86 per cent according to our clients' assessment, not ours [12].

So why is it that some nutritionists, doctors, scientists, politicians and food companies wish to lull us into a false sense of security by telling us that all we need to do is eat a 'well-balanced diet'? Why are we told that we don't need supplements, when in truth the majority of people do? Why are so many health professionals willing to deprive their patients of the potent and relatively safe approach of optimum nutrition?

Medical Schools Don't Teach Nutrition

I believe there are three reasons - ignorance, money and resistance to change. A doctor qualifying today is unlikely to have had as much as ten hours tuition in nutrition. Unless a doctor has pursued the study of nutrition out of choice he or she is unlikely to be sufficiently informed to advise about optimum nutrition. It is safer to give no advice or refer to someone who is informed, yet too many doctors advise people not to follow special diets or take supplements. This is especially dangerous during pregnancy since it is now well established that people who are vitamin or mineral deficient are more likely to have underweight babies or babies born with birth abnormalities[13]. Fortunately the British Society of Nutritional Medicine publishes a Journal and holds regular conferences to help doctors become informed about nutrition. Their address is given on page 158.

Nutritional Flat-Earthers

Then there are the flat-earthers who simply won't adjust to the wealth of new knowledge in this field. They argue that if you haven't got scurvy you've got enough vitamin C. If you eat a well-balanced diet you're not deficient. If a test result is normal you're healthy (even though you know you're not). They ignore the effects of pollution, drugs, disease and lifestyle on nutritional needs. Such fixed ideas are "adopted when a paradigm shift is occurring and the emergence of a new paradigm is 'generally preceded by a period of pronounced professional insecurity.' We are currently seeing a paradigm shift in the use of nutrition in the treatment and prevention of disease and sub-optimum function." says Dr Davies, chairman of the British Society of Nutritional Medicine [14].

The Politics of Nutrition

One big reason for hanging on to such out-dated beliefs is money. Before the law was passed enforcing the listing of additives on food packaging we were told they were quite safe. The cost to the food industry to make food without using these cheap chemicals was considerable. Although I hope few people really believe it, the sugar industry continue to tell us that sugar is good for you! The food industry makes money out of using cheap ingredients that don't go off and hopefully are addictive, such as sugar, chocolate and coffee. Did you know that not even a weevil can live off white flour? Can you imagine the financial implications for the food industry if suddenly foods were not allowed to be processed in such a way as to destroy nutrients? Or if the RDAs were doubled, showing just how deficient most foods are? Or if chemical and pesticide residues in food had to be declared? Vested interests do not support the public becoming informed about nutrition if it means you'll buy less of their product. Such vested interests influence us through advertising, the media and political lobbies. It is therefore important to know who the financial sponsors of any organisation are. If they are supported by companies who make money out of less nutritious foods their advice needs to be taken with caution. This applies to the British Nutrition Foundation which advises the government about nutritional policy, yet is itself funded by the major companies producing confectionery, high fat foods, processed meats, food chemicals and alcohol[15]. Within government itself many key MPs are also directors or consultants to major food and chemical companies[16].The Ministry of Agriculture, Food and Fisheries (MAFF), on the one hand, represent the food industry, and on the other, are responsible for many food issues that affect our health. In an ideal society we would insist on a separate ministry concerned with food and health issues which would not be subject to such conflicts of interest.

So who can you trust? The answer is your own body. If something makes sense, is supported by clear evidence and is safe then try it out and see how you feel. The proof, in nutrition, is in the eating. The following chapters tell you what is known about arthritis and diet, and how you may be able to help yourself through the food you eat.

7

The Detox Diet

There is one diet that has consistently worked for sufferers of arthritis, particularly rheumatoid arthritis. That is, not eating. Fasts, or modified fasts with fruit and vegetable juices has proven to be the most successful dietary strategy to date. Fasting has been shown to reduce most symptoms, subjectively and objectively, within days [17].

Since fasting is obviously not a long-term option what is it about fasting that produces such good results? Obviously the most likely explanation is that some food or drink is aggravating arthritis. There are many possible mechanisms currently being investigated to explain why many arthritis sufferers get better when avoiding certain foods or drinks. These include food allergies or intolerances, increased gut permeability, pathogens in the gut [18] and blood sugar imbalances.

Allergy is defined as an unusual reaction to a substance, whether drunk or eaten, inhaled or applied to the skin, that causes a reaction of the body's immune system. Since the whole process of inflammation is part of the body's immune reaction, and since there is so much evidence of abnormal immune responses in arthritis sufferers, an allergic reaction could easily encourage symptoms of arthritis. Food intolerance is a term applied to reactions that, as yet, have not been identified with abnormal immune reactions. How some substances aggravate arthritis is not yet known, yet many foods are known to cause symptoms of arthritis in susceptible people. (These are discussed in more detail later in this chapter.) Any arthritis sufferer needs to investigate whether or not they are susceptible to specific food allergies or intolerances, and eliminate the culprits.

Gut permeability varies from person to person. The gut wall must be permeable to an extent to allow key nutrients to pass through.

However most nutrients get in through carefully controlled 'doors'. Only specific guests are allowed through. For example, digested proteins, called amino acids, are carried through the gut wall. If a mineral has become bound to an amino acid then it too can pass. (This is called an amino acid chelated mineral.) Rheumatoid arthritis sufferers often have increased gut permeability, which may be made worse by NSAID medication[19]. This means that undigested material, bacteria or other substances in the gut may be able to pass through. The immune army goes on red alert to deal with the unwelcome guests, thereby encouraging immune reactions which also take place in the joints, causing inflammation. If the gut wall is excessively permeable, eating virtually any diet may make symptoms worse. Gut permeability can be caused by food allergies in the gut, which weaken the wall of the digestive tract, by the presence of undesirable organisms like bacteria or the fungus candida albicans, or by the lack of key nutrients, such as vitamins A,C and zinc, which are needed to keep the wall of the digestive tract strong and healthy.

Pathogens are undesirable organisms that can, and do reside in the guts of many people. We all have approximately three pounds of about 300 different strains of bacteria living within the gut. Some we could classify as good and others as bad, however the potentially 'bad' guys are not a hindrance as long as there are enough of the good guys around. These bacteria help us to digest food, fight off bad bacteria that enter the body, and they even make some vitamins. The presence of the wrong kind of bacteria, especially if the gut wall is permeable and they enter the blood stream, can cause ill-health. Since bacteria need food to survive, not eating reduces symptoms caused by bacterial imbalances. Another common pathogen in the gut is candida albicans. This is a yeast-like organism which, if it gets established in the gut, will put down roots into the gut wall and increase gut permeability. Sounds nasty doesn't it! Candida albicans infection is increasingly common, and once again, eating food, particularly sugary food, will aggravate this condition.

Based on the current evidence it is unlikely that the presence of pathogens is a major factor in the cause or symptoms in the majority of arthritis sufferers, however it is worth bearing these factors in mind.

Blood sugar imbalances are very common and may well affect arthritis symptoms. If you frequently consume sugar, sweet foods, alcohol, or stimulants such as tea, coffee, chocolate or cigarettes, you may be using these foods because of their blood sugar effect. If you are 'addicted' to any of these, in other words the thought of not having them for a month induces a state of panic, you are almost certainly using them to prop up your blood sugar levels. They are, however, more than likely to aggravate your arthritis. (This factor is discussed in detail in Chapter 9.)

Whether or not these factors are likely to apply to you can be tested by carrying out the 10 Day Detox Diet (see Chapter 23). This is designed to eliminate likely allergy provoking foods [20], reduce gut permeability, reduce reactions created by pathogenic organisms, and eliminate fast-releasing sugars and stimulants that upset blood sugar balance.

If you notice a definite improvement in some of your symptoms it is well worth your while making good use of this period of elimination and going on to test for potential allergy provoking foods. How you do this is explained in Chapter 26. If, on the other hand, this 10 Day Detox Diet makes no difference then follow the general anti-arthritis diet given in Chapter 24.

Breaking Your Addictions

The following tips on breaking your addictions will help you, not only during these ten days, but also afterwards because a high stimulant or sugar diet is definitely not recommended for arthritis or general health, whatever the outcome. I recommend you greatly reduce your intake of stimulants such as tea, coffee, sugar, chocolate and alcohol. Here are some tips to help you break your addictions.

Coffee contains three stimulants - caffeine, theobromine and theophylline. Although caffeine is the strongest, theophylline is known to disturb normal sleep patterns and theobromine has a similar effect to caffeine, although it is present in much smaller amounts in coffee. So decaffeinated coffee isn't stimulant free.

A high intake of coffee is definitely bad for you. High coffee consumers have a greater risk of cancer of the pancreas and a higher incidence of birth defects. Coffee also stops vital minerals being absorbed. The amount of iron absorbed is reduced to one third if coffee is drunk with a meal. Coffee promotes the excretion of calcium [21].

More controversial are the effects of small amounts of coffee. As a nutritionist I have seen many people cleared of minor health problems such as tiredness and headaches just from stopping drinking two or three coffees a day. Coffee may also increase pain. Animal studies have shown that both normal and decaffeinated coffee powders interfere with the brain's opiate receptors, which help relieve pain [22]. So avoiding coffee may increase your pain threshold.

The best way to find out what effect it has on you is to quit for a trial period of two weeks. You may get withdrawal symptoms for up to three days. These reflect how addicted you've become. After that, if you begin to feel perky and your health improves that's a good indication that you're better off without it. The most popular alternatives are Caro Extra, made with roasted barley, chicory and rye, dandelion coffee (Symingtons or Lanes) or herb teas. Caro is wheat-free, although severe grain allergics may still react. Most dandelion coffee contains lactose, derived from milk, which causes problems for some people with milk allergy.

Tea is the great British addiction. A strong cup of tea contains as much caffeine as a weak cup of coffee and is certainly addictive. Tea also contains tannin which interferes with the absorption of vital minerals such as iron and zinc. Like coffee, drinking too much tea is also associated with a number of health problems including an increased risk of stomach ulcers. It is likely that excessive tea drinking may increase gut permeability. Particularly addictive is Earl Grey tea containing bergamot, itself a stimulant. If you're addicted to tea and can't get going without a cuppa it may be time to stop for two weeks and see how you feel. The best tasting alternatives are Rooibosch tea (red bush tea) with milk or herb teas such as Blackcurrant Bracer or Red Zinger. Drinking very weak tea irregularly is unlikely to be a problem.

Sugar is perhaps the most common addiction of all. The more sweet foods you have the greater your taste for sweetness. We all have a natural sweet tooth which is nature's way of attracting animals to eat fruits. In nature, sweet foods are usually safe to eat. But by refining sugar we've learnt how to cheat nature and eat the pure stuff. Nowadays concentrated sugar comes in many disguises - glucose, such as Lucozade, malt, honey, syrups. All these help to develop a sweet tooth as do any food with concentrated sweetness, including grape juice or too much dried fruit such as raisins. However the sugar in most fruit, called fructose does not have the same effect on the body as glucose, malt or sucrose. Malt, which is derived from grains, and sucrose, or normal sugar, have both been shown to make arthritis symptoms worse on reintroduction in some people[23]. While too much sugar is associated with heart disease, diabetes, tooth decay and obesity, which will aggravate arthritis, sugar is addictive because of its effect on energy and mood. Eating concentrated sources of sugar increases your blood sugar level giving more mental and physical energy, at least in the short term. This is one cause for hyperactivity, both in children and adults. If you're not aware of this effect it is most noticeable if you stay off sugar for two weeks then have a sugar binge.

Frequent over-use of sugar can lead to glucose intolerance, which means an abnormal blood sugar balance. The symptoms may include irritability, aggressive outbursts, nervousness, depression, crying spells, dizziness, fears and anxiety, confusion, forgetfulness, inability to concentrate, fatigue, insomnia, headaches, palpitations, muscle cramps, excess sweating, digestive problems, allergies, blurred vision, excessive thirst and lack of sex drive. Does this sound like anyone you know? Probably three in every ten people have a mild form of glucose intolerance which, uncorrected, could lead to diabetes later in life.

Kicking the sugar habit takes time and perseverance. It is best to wean yourself off slowly since your taste buds get used to less and less sweetness. Stop adding sugar to cereals, or eating cereals containing sugar, and add fruit instead. When you want something sweet have a piece of fresh fruit. Get used to diluting fruit juices with water. Gradually decrease your overall intake of sweet foods. Once you're basically sugar-free the odd sweet food is no big deal.

Chocolate is full of sugar. It also contains cocoa as its major active ingredient. Cocoa provides significant quantities of the stimulant theobromine, whose action is similar although not as strong as caffeine. Theobromine is also obtained in cocoa drinks like hot chocolate. Being high in sugar and stimulants, plus its delicious taste, it's easy to become a chocaholic. The best way to quit the habit is to have one month with NO chocolate. Instead you can eat healthy 'sweets' from health food shops. My favourites are Sunflower bars and Karriba bars. After a month you will have lost the craving for chocolate.

Cola and some other fizzy drinks contain between 5 and 7mg of caffeine which is a quarter of that found in a weak cup of coffee. In addition, these drinks are often high in sugar and colourings and their net stimulant effect can be considerable. Check the ingredients list and stay away from drinks containing caffeine and chemical additives or colourings.

Alcohol is chemically very similar to sugar, and high in calories. It disturbs normal blood sugar balance and appetite. Enough alcohol suppresses appetite which leads to more 'empty' calories from alcohol and less nutritious calories from healthy food. Alcohol also destroys or prevents the absorption of many nutrients including vitamin C, B complex, calcium, magnesium and zinc. There is little doubt that alcohol often aggravates arthritis.

Choosing Alternatives

Bad habits are much easier to break if you have good alternatives to choose from. Nowadays there are many alternatives to tea, coffee, alcohol and chocolate. My favourites are Blackcurrant Bracer, Red Zinger, Caro Extra, Aqua Libra, and Sunflower bars. Try them out and find out what you like. You'll find them in most health food shops.

8

The Allergy Connection

Allergies are much more common than you think. In fact, almost one in every three people suffer from allergies - be it pollen, cats, 'housedust', foods, drugs or chemicals[23]. Among arthritis sufferers the incidence of allergies is likely to be much higher. But what exactly is an allergy?

To answer this question you need to know a bit about your body's army - the immune system. Inside your body is an army of immune cells on a 24 hour search and destroy mission. When they find an invader, like a virus, they destroy it. The main way the immune system captures its prey is by producing tailor made straight jackets for a particular invader, an 'antibody'. This is how vaccination works. The polio vaccine exposes your body to the polio virus, not enough to make you sick, but just enough for the immune army to make polio anti-bodies, which are there to protect you in the future. If you're allergic to pollen, when you breath in pollen, your body starts to produce anti-bodies to pollen, as the immune army moves in to kill.

The classic symptoms of an allergy include hay-fever, a stuffy and running nose, itchy eyes and skin, asthma, headaches, bloating, water retention and facial puffiness. These are the signs that your body is trying to get rid of something it doesn't like. Most allergic responses are of an inflammatory nature and can precipitate pain, swelling and stiffness in the joints and muscles.

Allergies to food are increasingly common. The most common offenders are dairy products and grains, in particular wheat, however many other foods cause reactions in some people. But why do some become allergic and others don't?

If, for some reason our digestive system isn't working so well, and we absorb into the body incompletely broken down foods, the immune army will treat this food as an invader and attack. Another reason for potential reactions is that the immune army is malnourished and hence over-reacts to harmless substances.

Food	Percent of Symptomatic Patients Affected by Food		
*Corn	56	Beef	32
**Wheat	54	Coffee	32
Bacon/Pork	39	Malt	27
Oranges	39	Cheese	24
Milk	37	Grapefruit	24
Oats	37	Tomato	22
Rye	34	Peanuts	20
Eggs	32	Sugar (cane)	20

* Corn is the most common in the US   ** Wheat is the most common in the UK

Data from L Darlington MD, FRCP in Rheumatic Disease Clinics of North America, Vol 17, No 2, May 1991

Figure 8 Foods Most Likely to Cause Allergy

Allergies are therefore much more likely to develop in those that have a weakened immune system, perhaps due, in part, to chronic inflammation, or poor digestion. The likely allergens are foods eaten frequently, especially those that are potentially irritable to the digestive system.

As far as arthritis is concerned the most likely suspects are grains and dairy products, followed by pork, beef and eggs.

Our Deadly Bread

Wheat, for example, is eaten by most people every day, with the average person eating between a quarter and half a pound in the form of bread, cakes, pasta and cereal. It contains a gastrointestinal irritant called gluten, and is Britain's number one allergen. Other grains like rye, barley and oats also contain gluten. These also cause allergic reactions in some people, as does corn (maize). Rice, buckwheat, millet and quinoa are unlikely to cause allergic reactions.

According to Dr Hicklin grains are the most common allergen in rheumatoid arthritis [24]. They put 22 patients onto a diet excluding likely allergy provoking foods. No less than 20 noted improvements in symptoms. When tested with different foods, 19 reported that specific foods made them worse, the most common being grains.

Gluten, according to Dr Nadya Coates, has a structure alien to the body's metabolism. It sticks to anything and encapsulates smaller molecules such as sugar, cholesterol, fats or minerals, which are then transported into the blood as such, inefficiently digested. Gluten, she believes, is the major interfering factor in all digestive processes, with wheat gluten being the most toxic of all. Gluten is, unquestionably, an intestinal irritant. In highly sensitive people the lining of the small intestine, which consists of small protrusions called villi, becomes flattened. This is known as coeliac disease and leads to malabsorption, diarrheoa and loss of weight. If you have any of the following symptoms, as well as joint pain or stiffness, a trial period off wheat, and possibly off all glutinous grains, is strongly recommended.

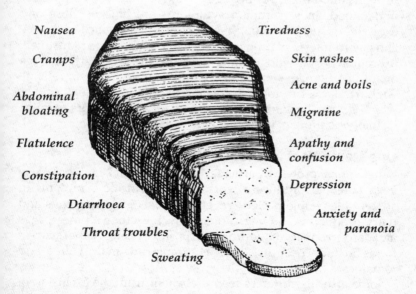

Nausea

Cramps

Abdominal bloating

Flatulence

Constipation

Diarrhoea

Throat troubles

Sweating

Tiredness

Skin rashes

Acne and boils

Migraine

Apathy and confusion

Depression

Anxiety and paranoia

Figure 9 *Symptoms Associated with Wheat and Gluten Sensitivity*

Milk and Allergy

Milk allergy or intolerance is very common in rheumatoid arthritis sufferers. Consider this case of a 52 year-old woman, reported by Dr Panush, Professor of medicine at the New Jersey Medical School, who went on a three day water fast, followed by a hypoallergenic (low allergy provoking) diet, excluding dairy produce[25]. Within 24 hours of starting the water fast there was noticeable symptomatic relief. She was then given encapsulated foods to test. There were no noticeable responses to 52 placebo challenges. On the four separate occasions she was given milk she reacted every time with a flare up of symptoms and a raised blood ESR, a measure of inflammation. Many similar reports of dairy allergy with arthritics have been published [26].

Sometimes reactions to dairy are a result of lactose intolerance since many adults lose the ability to digest lactose, milk sugar. The usual symptoms are bloating, abdominal pain, wind and diarrhoea, which subside on giving lactase, the enzyme that breaks down lactose. Probably equally common is an allergy or intolerance to proteins in dairy produce. For reasons not yet completely understood, most common symptoms are blocked nose and excessive mucus production, respiratory problems such as asthma, and gastro-intestinal problems. Such intolerances are more likely to occur in people who consume dairy products regularly, in large quantities. Some people who are intolerant to milk can tolerate yoghurt. Some can tolerate cow's milk or sheep's milk. Butter, which is virtually one hundred per cent fat and therefore contains virtually no protein, is less likely to cause a reaction.

One Man's Meat is Another Man's Poison

Other animal proteins, particularly pork, beef and eggs, have also been noted to produce a worsening of arthritic symptoms in susceptible people [27]. Both vegetarian diets including eggs and dairy products [28] and vegan diets, which exclude all meat, eggs and dairy produce [29] have produced positive results. Other suspect foods include peanuts, oranges, grapefruit, malt, coffee and tomatoes.

Some arthritis sufferers seem to benefit from the exclusion of foods in the nightshade family (solanaceae), which includes tomatoes, potatoes, aubergine, peppers and tobacco. This regime was made popular by a horticulturist called Childers, who found this simple exclusion to cure his arthritis[30]. Although unproven, these foods do contain solanum alkaloids which could theoretically inhibit normal collagen repair or promote inflammation.

While it is clear that many people do not show signs of allergies, many people, especially rheumatoid arthritics, do. The only way to find the best diet for you is to test for likely allergies.

Testing for Allergies

So how do you know if you've got an allergy and, if you have, what can you do about it? In truth it is not easy to know what you're allergic to. Any good nutritionist will investigate your allergic potential by looking at your diet and the kind of symptoms you have. If necessary they can run tests to check for allergies but no tests are one hundred per cent accurate. Ultimately, the best test is to avoid suspect foods and see how you feel. Once you know what you're reacting to, the best strategy is to avoid these substances for at least three months and meanwhile build up your immune system through a proper supplement programme. Once optimally nourished some people can tolerate small amounts of substances they used to react to.

Most people are free of symptoms within 10 to 20 days of avoiding an allergy provoking food. Most people react on reintroducing such a food within 48 hours, although some have a delayed reaction of up to 10 days. Delayed reactions are much harder to test. For some, symptoms improve considerably when leaving off offending foods. For others noticeable changes are hard to detect.

One simple way to help identify possible suspects is the pulse test, explained in Chapter 26. This is highly recommended for anyone who improves on the Detox Diet or who scores highly on the Allergy Test in Chapter 26. The pulse test requires avoiding all suspect foods for 20 days, then reintroducing them, one by one, with a 48 hour gap in between each item to be tested. Both changes in the pulse and symptoms are noted. If a food is reacted to, either by a marked increase in pulse rate, or by any symptoms, it is avoided before testing the next item.

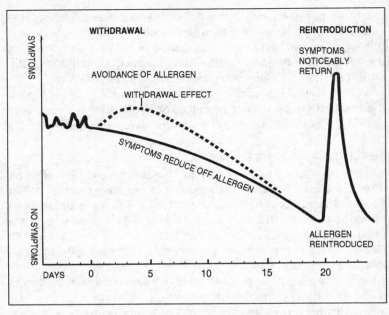

Figure 10 *The Avoidance/Reintroduction Test for Allergies*

While day to day changes in symptoms are hard to pin down to specific causes, avoidance of suspect foods for 20 days often lessens symptoms which then increase significantly on reintroduction. In this way it is often possible to notice which foods or drinks make you worse. It is very important to observe symptoms accurately because you may have preconceived ideas about what you do or don't react to, perhaps because of what somebody told you, including me, or because you dread being allergic to certain foods that you're addicted to.

9

The Anti-Arthritis Diet

The best kind of diet to combat arthritis is high in vitamins and minerals, sufficient and not excessive in protein, high in slow-releasing carbohydrate foods and low in fast-releasing sugar, high in essential fats and low in fat overall, and low in stimulants and alcohol. Certain foods have been noted as particularly beneficial for arthritis. Others may be better avoided, such as foods with a high allergenic potential, especially if allergy testing has confirmed that you react.

Balancing your Blood Sugar

Keeping your blood sugar level even is a critical factor for arthritis and overall health. Insulin, the major hormone released by the body to control blood sugar, stimulates the production and assembly of mucopolysaccharides into cartilage[31]. Diabetics, who have either deficiency of insulin or insensitivity to it, have more severe arthritis than non-diabetic arthritics[31,32]. Having an uneven blood sugar level also upsets calcium balance and is clearly a risk factor for arthritis. In addition, keeping your blood sugar balanced is probably the most important factor in weight control.

The level of glucose in your blood largely determines your appetite. When the level drops you feel hungry. When the levels are too high the body converts the excess to glycogen (a short term fuel store mainly in the liver and muscle cells) or fat, our long-term energy reserve. When the levels are too low we experience a whole host of symptoms including fatigue, poor concentration, irritability, nervousness, depression, excessive thirst, sweating, headaches and digestive problems. An estimated three in every ten people have glucose intolerance, an inability to keep an even blood sugar level. Their blood sugar level may go too high and then drop too low. The result, over the years, is that they become increasingly fat and lethargic. On the other hand, if you can control your blood sugar levels, the result is even weight and constant energy.

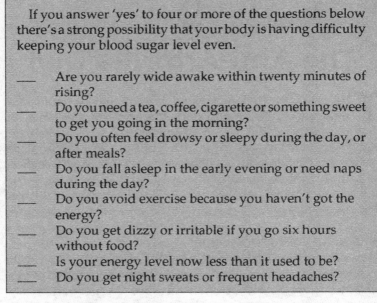

If you answer 'yes' to four or more of the questions below there's a strong possibility that your body is having difficulty keeping your blood sugar level even.

_____ Are you rarely wide awake within twenty minutes of rising?

_____ Do you need a tea, coffee, cigarette or something sweet to get you going in the morning?

_____ Do you often feel drowsy or sleepy during the day, or after meals?

_____ Do you fall asleep in the early evening or need naps during the day?

_____ Do you avoid exercise because you haven't got the energy?

_____ Do you get dizzy or irritable if you go six hours without food?

_____ Is your energy level now less than it used to be?

_____ Do you get night sweats or frequent headaches?

Figure 11 Glucose Tolerance Check

So what makes your blood sugar level unbalanced? Obviously eating too much sugar and sweet foods. However, the kind of foods that have the greatest effect are not always what you might expect. Figure 13 on page 64 shows which foods have the most profound effect on blood sugar levels. The worst is glucose which is the simplest form of sugar. Malt sugar, Lucozade and Mars Bars all contain glucose, as does most honey. Fructose, the sugar in fruit, has little effect.

Of the fruits, bananas and dried fruit has the greatest effect on blood sugar, and apples have the least. Whole grains have a small effect on blood sugar, unless they are refined. Commercial bread, brown or white, white rice and white pasta all have increased effects compared to their whole counterparts. The best bread is Scandinavian whole rye grain bread, such as Pumpernickel bread. Oatcakes also have a small effect on blood sugar. Cornflakes came out badly for breakfast cereals, with porridge oats being the best.

The best foods of all are pulses - peas, beans and lentils. None of these have substantial effects on blood sugar. Milk products, which contain the sugar lactose, are also good. Surprisingly, even ice-cream comes out well. But don't kid yourself - it's still high in fat, even if it doesn't alter blood sugar levels much.

Vegetables, when cooked or highly processed, can have a considerable effect on blood sugar. Instant mashed potato has as strong an effect as a Mars Bar. Carrots and parsnips are the sweetest vegetables, however, if eaten raw or lightly cooked, have a much less dramatic effect.

Alcohol, which is a chemical cousin of sugar, also upsets blood sugar levels. So do stimulants, like tea, coffee, cola drinks, and cigarettes. These substances, like stress itself, stimulate the release of adrenalin and other hormones that initiate the "fight or flight" response. This prepares the body for action, by releasing sugar stores and raising blood sugar levels, to give our muscles and

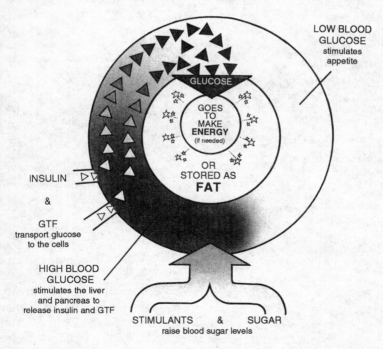

Figure 12 The Sugar Cycle

Which Foods Raise Blood Sugar Levels?

The foods with the great effect on blood sugar have the highest score.

Sugars

Glucose	100
Maltose	100
Lucozade	95
Honey	87
Mars Bar	68
Sucrose (sugar)	59
Fructose	20

Fruit

Raisins	64
Bananas	62
Orange juice	46
Oranges	40
Apples	39

Grain Products

Brown bread	72
White rice	72
White bread	69
Ryvita	69
Brown rice	66
Pastry	59
Digestive biscuits	59
Sweetcorn	59
Rich tea biscuits	55
Oatmeal biscuits	54
White spaghetti	50
Wholemeal spaghetti	42

Cereals

Cornflakes	80
Weetabix	75
Shredded wheat	67
Muesli	66
All-Bran	52
Porridge oats	49

Pulses

Baked beans (no sugar)	40
Butter beans	36
Chick peas	36
Blackeye beans	33
Haricot beans	31
Kidney beans	29
Lentils	29
Soya beans	15

Dairy Products

Ice cream	36
Yoghurt	36
Whole milk	34
Skimmed milk	32

Vegetables

Cooked parsnips	97
Cooked carrots	92
Instant potato	80
New potato	70
Cooked beetroot	64
Peas	51

Figure 13 Glyceamic Index of Foods

brains a boost of energy. Unlike our ancestors whose main stresses (like running up a tree to avoid being eaten for dinner) required a physical response, twentieth century stress is mainly mental or emotional. The body has to cope with the excess of blood sugar by releasing yet more hormones to take the glucose out of circulation. The combination of too much sugar, stimulants and prolonged stress taxes the body and results in an inability to control blood sugar levels, which, if severe enough, can develop into diabetes.

The only way out of this vicious cycle is to reduce or avoid all forms of concentrated sweetness, tea, coffee, alcohol and cigarettes, and start eating foods that help to keep your blood sugar level even. The best foods are all kinds of beans, peas and lentils, oats and wholegrains. These foods are high in complex carbohydrates and contain special factors that help release their sugar content gradually. They are also high in fibre which helps normalise blood sugar levels.

Protein Myths

What words do you associate with protein? Meat, eggs, cheese, muscles, growth. You have to eat these foods to get enough protein to grow big and strong. Right?... or wrong?

The word protein is derived from 'protos', meaning 'first' since protein is the basic material of all living cells. The human body is, for example, approximately 65% water and 25% protein. Protein is made out of amino acids, building blocks of nitrogen-containing molecules. Some 23 different types of amino acids are pieced together in different combinations to make different kinds of protein, which form the material for our cells and organs, in much the same way as letters make words, which combine to make sentences and paragraphs.

From eight basic amino acids, the remaining 16 can be made. These eight are termed essential amino acids, although others are semi-essential under certain conditions. The body cannot function without any one of these eight. Each one deserves its own 'recommended intake' although these have yet to be set. The balance of these eight amino acids in the protein of any given food determines its quality, or usability. So, how much protein do you need and what is the best quality protein?

Estimates for protein requirement vary enormously depending on who you speak to. This is not so surprising since there may be widespread 'biochemical individuality'. At the low end of the scale are reports of protein sufficiency when 2.5% of total calorie intake comes from protein. The World Health Organisation recommends 4.5% of total calories from protein, while the US National Research Council adds on a safety margin and recommends 8% as adequate for 95% of the population. Human breast milk, sufficient for the rapid growth of infants, derives 5% of calories from protein. The World Health Organisation suggests that an infant needs relatively twice as much protein as an adult, so it is certainly unlikely than an adult would require much more than 5% of total calories from protein. This equates to roughly 30 to 40 grams of protein for the average adult male. The estimated average requirement per day, according to the Department of Health, is 36g for women and 44g for men. If the quality of protein eaten is high, less protein needs to be eaten.

So, which foods provide more than 5% of calories from protein? You may be surprised to find that virtually every single lentil, bean, vegetable, nut, seed, grain and most fruits provide more than 5% protein. 54% of calories in soya beans come from protein, compared to 26% in a kidney bean. Spinach is 49% protein, while a potato is only 11%. Grains vary from 16% for quinoa to 4% for corn. Nuts and seeds range from 21% for pumpkin seeds to 12% for cashews. Fruit varies from 16% for lemons down to 1% for apples. What this means in real terms is that if someone is eating enough calories they are almost certainly eating enough protein, unless they are living off junk food, high in sugar and fat.

This may come as a surprise, to cut against the grain of all we are taught about protein. Yet the fact of the matter is, to quote a team of Harvard scientists investigating vegetarian diets, "It is difficult to obtain a mixed vegetable diet which will produce an appreciable loss of body protein." But isn't animal protein better quality than plant protein?

Animal or Vegetable?

Once again, there are a few surprises. Top of the class is quinoa, a high protein grain from South America that was a staple food

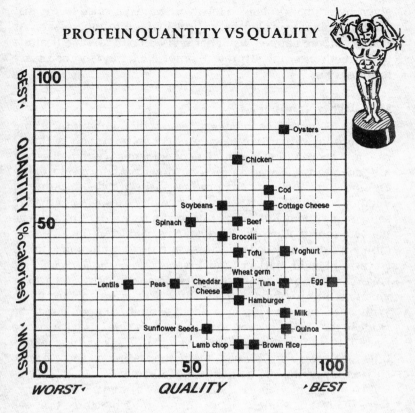

Figure 14 Quality and Quantity of Protein in Foods

during the Inca empire. Quinoa has a quality of protein better than meat. So too does soya. Most vegetables are relatively low in the amino acids methionine and lysine, however beans and lentils are rich in methionine. Soya beans and quinoa are excellent sources of both lysine and methionine. Vegetarians are also less prone to osteoporosis than meat eaters[33] and lose less calcium from bones than meat eaters between the critical ages of 30 and 60 [34].

Early theories, such as those first expounded by Frances Moore Lappe, suggested that vegetable proteins had to be carefully combined with complementary proteins to match the quality given by animal proteins. However, we have since learnt that careful combining of plant based proteins is quite unnecessary. As Frances Moore Lappe says in her revised book "With a healthy, varied diet, concern about protein complementarity is not necessary for most of us."

Milk - Who Needs It?

Not only is it possible to have a healthy diet without including dairy produce, excessive dairy product consumption is almost certainly contributing to a number of epidemic western diseases. My general advice for anyone is to cut down on dairy produce. The arguments in favour of dairy produce are its protein, calcium and vitamin content. There are, however, many excellent alternative sources of protein. Regarding calcium, dairy produce may not be the best source after all. Good sources of calcium include nuts (almonds, brazils), seeds (sesame, sunflower, pumpkin), pulses (soya flour, tofu, haricot beans), vegetables (spinach, cabbage, kale, carrots), and fruits (apricots, figs, rhubarb). Regarding vitamins, milk is a good source of vitamin D, as are eggs and meat. With sufficient exposure to sunlight enough vitamin D may be made in the skin, however, to be on the safe side it is wise to take a multivitamin containing 400ius of vitamin D if your diet contains little meat, fish, eggs or milk. Many foods designed for vegans, such as soya milk, also contain added vitamin D.

A comparison of human milk with cow's or goat's milk shows three interesting things. Firstly, human milk has three times as much protein as well as substantially more calcium. Secondly, cow's milk has a higher phosphorus to calcium ratio. This is also relevant because in animals a relatively high intake of phosphorus to calcium induces osteoporosis. Calcium and phosphorus have a complicated relationship. Calcium and phosphorus are bound together in bone. When calcium is released into the blood, phosphorus is also released, only to be excreted via the kidneys. A high dietary phosphorus intake may render less 'free' calcium available for buffering an over-acidic blood, hence effectively inducing calcium deficiency.

While the UK represents 20% of the EC population, it consumes 40% of its dairy produce. Drinking milk and eating dairy products in our current excessive quantities does not, however, seem to be preventing osteoporosis. Since excessive protein consumption is a risk factor for developing osteoporosis, increasing dairy products, a major source of protein in the average diet, may not be the best way of ensuring adequate calcium intake.

The Fats of Life

Two people with rheumatoid arthritis obtained relief in days, which lasted for 9 and 14 months respectively, by going on a low-fat diet. Within 48 hours of eating a high fat diet they experienced their old symptoms again[35]. These observations have been reported by other rheumatoid arthritis sufferers and suggest that the effect of a low fat diet is far more than simple weight reduction which would be expected to reduce arthritic symptoms in the long-term, not within 48 hours. One possible explanation could be that diets containing saturated fat block the conversion of essential fatty acids into anti-inflammatory prostaglandins. By removing all fat, anti-inflammatory prostaglandin activity may be improved.

While I recommend a low fat diet I do not recommend a no fat diet. In view of the importance of essential fatty acids found in fish, nuts, seeds and their oil, the ideal anti-arthritis diet should be very low in saturated fat, and sufficient in these essential fatty acids. In practical terms this means eating more vegetarian foods and less animal products since most of our saturated fat comes from meat, eggs and dairy produce.

A vegan diet, which means no meat, fish, eggs and dairy produce, is a guaranteed way to reduce saturated fat. As long as seeds and nuts, or their oils are included, a vegan diet should encourage the body to produce anti-inflammatory prostaglandins, which may explain the results of the following study. Twenty rheumatoid arthritis sufferers went on a vegan diet which also excluded coffee, tea, sugar, alcohol, salt and strong spices. After four months 12 reported feeling better, 5 reported no change and 3 felt worse. Most felt less pain and were better able to function, although objective measures of grip strength didn't change[36]. (Of course, it is always hard to know whether these patients would have been expected to get worse over four months anyway.)

Is Your Weight A Burning Issue?

There is little doubt that excess weight makes arthritis worse and joint damage more likely. Obesity has been associated with both osteo and rheumatoid arthritis, particularly in weight bearing joints. A recent survey of 4,225 people with osteoarthritis found that obesity was definitely associated with osteoarthritis in the knees, particularly among women[37]. Physical examination of obese people found evidence of osteoarthritis in the knee even in people who had no evidence of knee pain. Frame size made little difference.

While the mechanical stress of excess weight on joints seems to be the major reason for the association between obesity and arthritis, other researchers have reported an association between obesity and arthritis in non-weight bearing joints, such as fingers[38]. This suggests a systemic imbalance, probably of the endocrine system, that connects weight and joint problems.

Many people with weight problems also have a sluggish metabolism probably due to glucose intolerance, itself the result of excessive stress, sugar and stimulants. As well as paving the way for obesity this syndrome is likely to disturb the balance of hormones controlling calcium levels in bone. It is more than likely that diet is the link between obesity and arthritis.

Whichever comes first, obesity or arthritis, once movement and therefore exercise is restricted it becomes harder to lose weight. Highly restrictive diets are unlikely to provide optimum amounts of all the nutrients that may lessen arthritis symptoms. However, by following the diet recommended in this book, which is designed to improve your metabolism and keep your blood sugar level even, weight can be lost without severe calorie restriction. The Sunday Times reported greater weight loss on the Fatburner Diet (see page 151 for details on this book) supplying 1,500 calories than on the Cambridge Diet supplying 330 calories.

So, if you are overweight, follow the recommendations of this diet strictly, reducing quantities as needed, and stick to a regular exercise regime which burns calories while not overstraining the joints. My book, The Fatburner Diet, gives such a diet and exercise programme that is consistent with an anti-arthritis regime (see page 151 for details).

Beneficial Foods

The vast majority of the vitamins and minerals we need come from vegetables and fruit. These food groups should make up 50% of the food we eat. This means eating like a rabbit - three pieces of fruit a day and large amounts of vegetables with meals. Most vegetables are best eaten raw, or lightly cooked (steaming is best).

Cherries, blueberries and hawthorn berries and their juice are good for gout because they contain anthocyanidins and proanthocyanadins which are types of flavanoids giving these foods their deep red-blue colour. They have been shown to help enhance collagen matrix integrity and to have anti-inflammatory effects [39]. Quercitin, discussed in the Appendix on page 150, is another example of a naturally occurring flavanoid with anti-inflammatory properties.

Onions and garlic are rich in sulphur containing amino acids, cystine and methionine. These amino acids are essential constituents in both cartilage and anti-oxidant enzymes and are likely to be of benefit. There is some evidence that sulphur itself may benefit arthritis [40]. Most hot springs contain water rich in sulphur, which is absorbed into the body, perhaps being one of the reasons for the reputed benefits of these remedial baths [41]. Eggs are also a rich source of sulphur containing amino acids, however too many eggs are not recommended due to their high fat content and the fact that some people are allergic to them. The kind of fat in an egg depends very much on the feed the chicken has been given. If the feed is rich in essential fatty acids then so too is the egg. Therefore it is best to eat genuinely free-range eggs, and not to fry them to minimise free radicals.

Part 3

Vitamins, Minerals & Arthritis

10

The Benefits of B Vitamins

The group of B vitamins are among the most essential nutrients for health. Since they do not store in the body a daily supply is necessary for energy production, healthy nerves, skin and a host of other key roles including hormone and prostaglandin production and balance, a vital factor in arthritic diseases. One B vitamin is directly involved in the production of cortisone. Vitamin B5 is also called pantothenic acid, from the Greek word 'pantos' meaning everywhere, because it is found in so many foods. Despite this many people do not get enough of this essential nutrient, which is also needed to make energy in every single cell, and helps make acetylcholine, an important chemical in the brain that is thought to be involved in memory.

Pantothenic acid (Vitamin B5)

As long ago as 1950 it was known that animals severely deficient in pantothenic acid developed osteoarthritis, including osteoporosis, calcification of cartilage and the formation of osteophytes [1]. This led Dr Annand in Dundee to experiment with giving his osteoarthritic patients pantothenic acid [2]. He found that a supplement of 12.5mg each morning and evening produced an improvement in their condition, as well as a drop in ESR. Improvement did not manifest for 7 to 10 days. On stopping supplementation symptoms once again returned.

Particularly lacking in this B vitamin are rheumatoid arthritics. A study of 66 arthritis patients found their blood levels of pantothenic acid to be very much lower than those without arthritis [3]. This study also found that vegetarians tended to have higher levels than those eating a 'normal' diet. This is not surprising since vegetables are a good source of pantothenic acid.

Could pantothenic acid also help rheumatoid arthritis sufferers?

The researchers decided to test this theory by giving 20 rheumatoid arthritis patients with low pantothenic acid levels, injections of pantothenic acid for a month. Within seven days both symptoms and blood levels of pantothenic acid had improved. Once the intravenous pantothenic acid was stopped, blood levels again dropped and symptoms returned [3].

This study was repeated under more rigorous conditions 17 years later, using supplements instead of injections [4]. Eighteen rheumatoid arthritis patients were given either 500mg of pantothenic acid four times a day (as calcium pantothenate) or a placebo. After two months there was a reduction in morning stiffness, severity of pain and disability.

Exactly how pantothenic acid works is still a bit of a mystery. It is required for the production of corticosteroids, the body's natural anti-inflammatory agents. This may explain the improvement in rheumatoid arthritis, however the formation of osteoarthritis-like joint changes seen in deficient animals suggests a role in joint health, perhaps through affecting calcium balance.

Meanwhile, pantothenic acid is certainly worth trying for any form of arthritis. I know of no trials to date using significant amounts of pantothenic acid which have failed to show a positive response. I recommend 500 to 1,000mg of pantothenic acid for any arthritis sufferer for a trial period of a month. Pantothenic acid supplementation may also help gout, which is a build up of uric acid in the body, since it helps convert uric acid to urea and ammonia which can be eliminated from the body.

Vitamin B3 - Niacinamide

Another B vitamin that has proven helpful for arthritics is vitamin B3, known as niacin or niacinamide. Niacinamide has been used with good results since 1943. It is interesting to note, in a letter from Dr William Kaufman, who pioneered this research, of the similar resistance to nutritional therapy encountered today compared to that of more than 40 years ago. "Ever since 1943 I have tried to call my work on niacinamide to the attention of leading rheumatologists, nutritionists and gerontologists through conversations with them, by sending them copies of my monographs and papers on this subject, and by two talks given on the usefulness of niacinamide and other vitamins which I gave at the International Gerontological Congresses in 1951 and 1954. I think that two factors have made it difficult for doctors to accept the concept that continuous therapy with large doses of niacinamide could cause improvement in joint dysfunction and give other benefits: (a) the advent of cortisone, and (b) the fact that my use of vitamins was such a departure from the recommended daily allowance for vitamins by the National Research Council."

The recipient of this letter, Dr Abram Hoffer, had contacted Dr Kaufman after coincidentally finding that some of his patients whom he was treating with high doses of niacin, either for schizophrenia or for high cholesterol levels, were reporting improvement in their arthritis [5]. He reported six cases of osteo and rheumatoid arthritis who received either niacin or niacinamide in doses of 1,000 to 3,000mg per day, four of whom effected a complete recovery, one of whom was described as 'nearly normal', and the last as much improved. Here is one excerpt from the case of Mrs HC, who was diagnosed with osteoarthritis at the age of 68 in February 1954. "Her hands were becoming deformed and showed marked ulnar deviation, well-marked Heberden's nodes on all fingers, and severe pain on movement. In March 1954, she was started on 1 gram niacin per day in two divided doses. She has continued on this medication until the present report (1959). About three months later (July 1954) I again examined the patient. There was a marked improvement, mentally and physically. She no longer complained of neuritis; her vision became normal and has not failed her since. The ulnar deviation of her hands vanished, as did the Heberden's nodes. These nodes went through an interesting change. In random order they first enlarged somewhat, then receded in size until they became hardly visible. Her hands became normally mobile. The skin regained its previous elasticity and tone."

Dr William Kaufman who pioneered the use of vitamin B3 as niacinamide, devised a simple, objective method for determining joint mobility, and set to work recording the effects of niacinamide therapy, which he gave in doses of 900 to 4,000mg per day, in divided doses with or without other vitamins. By 1955 he had recorded the effects of niacinamide on 663 patients [6]. He showed conclusively that, without exception, patients who took adequate amounts of niacinamide on a continuous basis had significant and measurable improvement in joint mobility and function, less stiffness, less joint deformity and lowered ESR levels. These results were seen in rheumatoid and osteoarthritis sufferers and continued as long as the supplementation was continued. Removal of supplementation resulted in worsening of symptoms.

How Much Is Safe?

The niacin form of vitamin B3, which is the most effective for lowering high cholesterol levels, causes a blushing sensation. This usually last for up to 30 minutes and is not harmful, although some people find it unpleasant. Niacin can produce adverse reactions at levels above 3,000mg per day. Sustained release has even greater toxicity and is not recommended.

The niacinamide form, which is the preferred form for arthritis, does not cause a blushing effect. While I am unaware of any reports of toxicity of niacinamide at the levels used by Dr Kaufman I would not recommend supplementing more than 1,000mg per day of either niacin or niacinamide unless under the guidance and supervision of a doctor or nutritionist. This level, however, would appear to be entirely safe [7].

B6 - Pyridoxine

Another vitamin that relieves symptoms of arthritis is pyridoxine, vitamin B6. Dr John Ellis from Mount Pleasant in Texas found that giving B6 in doses of 50mg helped to control pain and restored joint mobility to his patients [8]. Vitamin B6 shrinks the synovial membranes that line the bearing surfaces of the joints. It also helps to regulate the synthesis of anti-inflammatory prostaglandins.

Dr Ellis also found another use for this vitamin in the relief of a nerve disorder called carpal tunnel syndrome. This is a painful and crippling disease affecting the hands and wrists caused by compression of the principal nerve supply for the hand as it passes through a tunnel lined with *synovial membrane* between the tendons and ligaments in the wrist. A double-blind controlled study by Ellis and Karl Folkers [9], proved that B6 was so effective that, "pyridoxine therapy may frequently obviate hand surgery."

11

The Free Radical Fighters - Selenium, C and E

One of the major causes of cell damage is the behaviour of free radicals. A free radical is an atom or group of atoms with an uneven electrical charge. To complete itself it steals a charged particle (an electron) from a neighbouring cell, which can set up a chain of reactions producing more free radicals, damaging more cells and causing them to misbehave. Many normal chemical reactions, such as breathing in oxygen and turning it into carbon dioxide, give rise to the formation of free radicals. Unsaturated oils, such as vegetable oils, are particularly susceptible to free radical damage, especially when heated. So we have developed ways of dealing with these by-products of using oxygen, through anti-oxidation.

Anti-oxidant nutrients play an important role in inflammation. Anti-oxidants, like vitamin C and vitamin E, protect our cells from free radical attack and reduce inflammation. Both have been shown to increase lifespan [10]. Nuts and seeds also contain vitamin E to protect their essential oils from oxidation, which is the same as rancidity. Yet some oil manufacturers remove vitamin E and sell us vegetable oil that is prone to rancidity.

We also have enzymes designed to disarm free radicals. One of these, SOD (superoxide dismutase), is at the forefront of arthritis research, which has led to the sale of SOD tablets in health food shops. Yet there is little evidence that SOD taken in tablets can survive the perils of digestion and remain intact to strengthen us from the damaging effect of oxides. One type of SOD depends on a careful balance of copper and zinc. An excess or deficiency of copper or zinc have also been shown to be associated with worsening symptoms of arthritis. Another type of SOD depends

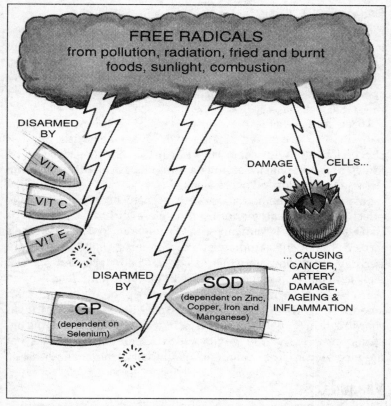

Figure 15 *Anti-Oxidant Nutrients and Sources of Free Oxidising Radicals*

on iron. Once again, excesses and deficiencies are associated with worsening symptoms. Yet another type of SOD depends on manganese, deficiency of which is known to result in cartilage problems in joints.

A close relative anti-oxidant enzyme, GP (glutathione peroxidase), depends on the mineral selenium. Increase the dietary intake of selenium by a factor of ten and you will double the activity of GP[11]. In both animals and man high selenium is associated with low risk of cancer.

Selenium

Forty years ago selenium was known only as a toxic mineral. Now it is recognised as one of the most essential trace elements for man. Deficiency of this element increases the risk of cancer, heart disease and arthritis. US and UK governments are currently sponsoring research to find out just how much we need to prevent these major diseases.

Three studies have found low levels of selenium in arthritic patients [12]. One checked 26 girls with juvenile arthritis, another checked adults with rheumatoid arthritis. Levels tended to be lowest in people with the severest symptoms. Levels of the selenium dependent enzyme GP were also low.

Selenium supplementation has recently been shown to be effective in the treatment of rheumatoid arthritis [13]. Dr Peretz, at the Department of Rheumatology at Brugmann Hospital in Brussels gave eight patients supplements containing 200mcg of selenium per day, and compared them to seven patients given placebo supplements. According to Dr Peretz "pain and joint involvement were reduced in most (six out of eight) patients treated with selenium while the placebo group showed no significant modification." In his opinion selenium probably works by stimulating GP enzyme activity which detoxifies free radicals that are generated in large amounts in inflammatory rheumatic diseases.

Vitamin C & E

Vitamin C has been found to be low in rheumatoid arthritis sufferers [14], quite possibly due to the degree of inflammation, which increases free radical activity within the affected area. Being a free radical scavenger vitamin C sacrifices itself in the process of fighting free radicals.

But vitamin C is not only an anti-oxidant. It is also necessary for cartilage and bone formation. Collagen cannot be synthesised without vitamin C. Deficiency causes severe signs of osteoarthritis in guinea pigs, who, like us are not able to synthesize their own vitamin C [15]. Guinea pigs given sufficient amounts of vitamin C do not develop osteoarthritis. Both vitamin C and E help to control the synthesis of mucopolysaccharides which help the formation of cartilage. As long ago as 1964 vitamin C was found to relieve back pain possibly by helping to preserve disc integrity[16]. More recently there have been reports of positive results using 'Ester-C', a vitamin C product that contains the metabolites produced from vitamin C. There is some evidence that these metabolites may be much more effective than vitamin C itself. Dr Edwin Goertz, a Canadian physician, has used Ester-C with 300 patients with good results: "At least 5 per cent have reported good results in their symptoms using Ester-C either as a primary treatment or as an adjunctive therapy"[17].

Since vitamin C is a water soluble anti-oxidant and vitamin E is a fat soluble anti-oxidant, protecting fatty layers of cells, the combination of these two nutrients may well help reduce inflammation and speed up healing of joints. The recommended intake of vitamin E is up to 500ius per day, while the recommended intake of vitamin C is from 3 to 10 grams per day.

The Value of Vitamin E

Vitamin E is a valuable allay in the fight against inflammation. There is little question that vitamin E deficiency increases free radical activity within joints[18], and that supplementing vitamin E reduces this potential cause of inflammation[19]. In animals a lack of vitamin E causes arthritis, which can be reversed by ensuring optimal intakes of this vital anti-oxidant[20]. Government backed research is currently investigating how strong this effect is in people with inflammatory joint diseases such as arthritis[21]. According to research in the USA many arthritis sufferers may not get anywhere near enough vitamin E to limit inflammation[22]. In a diet survey, 20 out of 24 rheumatoid arthritis sufferers and 11 out of 12 osteoarthritis sufferers consumed less than half the RDA for vitamin E. Intakes of vitamin E in the order of 600ius per day have been shown to help arthritis sufferers. Due to its anti-inflammatory role by preventing free radical damage to joint tissue one would expect vitamin E to be most important in rheumatoid arthritis.

12

Iron - Do We Really need Extra?

Nowadays many supplements as well as drinks, bread and breakfast cereals sell themselves on the 'extra added iron'. But do we really need this much? Iron is concentrated in the blood, and is found in every cell in our bodies. Iron's main function is to help carry oxygen to all cells. Without oxygen nothing would happen, so it's a vital function. This it does by combining with protein and copper to make red blood cells that transport oxygen to each cell. Iron is also needed for the anti-oxidant enzyme SOD to work. For this reason having sufficient iron is especially important if you're suffering from an inflammatory disease like arthritis. Although many vegetarian foods contain iron, like beans, lentils, wholegrains, wheatgerm, apricots and eggs, the iron in meat is much more absorbable. Eating vitamin C rich foods with vegetarian sources of iron increases the amount of iron absorbed. So scrambled eggs on wholegrain toast with a glass of orange juice would deliver significant amounts of iron.

Iron is one of the few minerals doctors are all to keen to prescribe, especially for women during pregnancy. While it is true that around one in ten people are iron deficient too much iron can also be bad. Once again, it's all a question of balance because very high levels of iron can induce zinc deficiency. In practical terms it is not wise to supplement more than 15mg of iron unless a test has been run to determine a person is definitely iron deficient, and extra zinc is given as well.

Iron levels in the joints and synovial fluid of arthritis sufferers are usually considerably higher than those without arthritis[23]. This is thought to indicate that iron, as part of the anti-oxidant army against inflammation and joint damage, is needed in larger amounts. Levels in the blood are usually low, possibly indicating that on-going inflammation uses up iron reserves. In most cases, when a bout of inflammation is over, synovial iron levels decrease and blood levels increase.

One study in which iron was supplemented had positive results[24]. However, for some people supplementation of substantial levels of iron may be unwise. One woman, diagnosed as iron deficient, supplemented her diet and, within three days her arthritis symptoms were much worse. Off the iron supplements she got better, on them she got worse [25]. Another patient, diagnosed as iron deficient, had relief of iron deficiency symptoms, but then went on to develop severe rheumatoid arthritis within two weeks. On investigation her hands and feet showed long-term erosive changes consistent with rheumatoid arthritis, but, up until that time she had had no symptoms, no pain, until she took the iron [26].

There are two possible explanations for these unusual stories. The first is that iron is needed for the body's normal inflammatory responses, probably as part of SOD, the anti-oxidant enzyme. In cases of iron deficiency the body is unable to respond in the normal way, hence no pain, although the joint degeneration clearly was taking place. Once the iron deficiency was corrected, inflammation started. There may be an element of truth in this theory, but one would not expect excessive inflammation.

The other possible, and perhaps more plausible explanation is this. Free radicals are dangerous oxides that damage joint tissue. In order to disarm the free radical it must first be acted on by the enzyme SOD, dependent on iron. This does not actually disarm the free radical. It is still dangerous, however it is now in a form that can be disarmed by its partner GP (glutathione peroxidase). GP is dependent on selenium.

If you give someone extra iron in an active stage of inflammation this could, in fact, increase free radical activitity [27]. Presumably, if you gave a sufficient amount of selenium this would minimise this possibility.

What we can conclude at this point in time is that there are potential dangers with overprescribing iron, and potential benefits, for some arthritic patients. It may be far safer to give an all-round multimineral supplement containing zinc, manganese, selenium and small amounts of iron, and copper to maintain the right balance of these essential trace elements.

13
The Zinc Link

Zinc, like iron, is part of the anti-oxidant enzyme SOD, and involved in inflammation. Like iron, high levels tend to be found in the synovial fluid of arthritics[28], while other body indicators show low or deficient levels. The assumption here is that zinc is used up at a faster rate when there is an on-going active inflammatory disease such as arthritis. Zinc is vital for hundreds of enzymes in the body, especially in relation to healthy immune function, growth, repair and protein utilisation. So, theoretically, adequate zinc should be essential for cartilage repair, proper immune and inflammatory responses, and warding off viruses and other infections.

Zinc is not only theoretically good for arthritis, it has proven beneficial in a research trial at the Division of Rheumatology, University of Washington [29]. Twenty four patients with chronic rheumatoid arthritis were given 50mg of zinc three times a day or an identical dummy pill for twelve weeks. At the end of twelve weeks all patients were given zinc. During the first twelve week period those who took zinc had less joint swelling, less morning stiffness, could walk further and generally felt better than those on the dummy pills. When those previously taking the dummy pills started taking zinc they too improved.

This trial was repeated with a group of psoriatic arthritics, again with positive results[30]. The most significant results, which included less joint pain and less morning stiffness, were seen after 5 weeks on zinc. These improvements were accompanied by a reduction in serum immunoglobulins, which suggested a less 'reactive' immune system in these patients following zinc supplementation.

However, a third trial using the same amount of zinc in severe long-standing rheumatoid arthritis sufferers found improvement in only 6 out of 22 patients [31].

Zinc is also vital for proper digestion. Protein cannot be digested without the combination of hydrochloric acid in the stomach and protein digesting enzymes. The production of both of these substances depends on zinc. So zinc deficiency could lead to poor protein digestion, paving the way for gut reactions to undigested proteins, possibly precipitating food allergies which encourage joint inflammation. There is evidence that arthritics may produce insufficient amounts of hydrochloric acid [32].

Zinc is not only vital for us it's vital for plants too. That's why all nuts, seeds and the germ of grains, such as wheat or oat germ, are all good sources of zinc. Animal produce also supplies zinc since zinc is required for the development of all new cells. The richest known sourc of zinc is oysters. Refined food has virtually no zinc and most vegetables and fruit contain little, unless you eat the seeds. Sesame seeds and sunflower seeds are good sources of zinc because they also contain calcium, magnesium, selenium and vitamin E. I have a spoonful of either sunflower seeds or ground sesame seeds every day.

Zinc is probably the most common mineral we lack in Britain. The average intake of zinc is around 8mg a day, which falls along way short of the World Health Organisation's recommended intake of 15mg a day. Someone with ongoing inflammation may need up to 25mg a day. With the right kind of diet you can guarantee an intake of 10 to 15mg a day, leaving a possible deficit of up to 15mg a day. That is why I recommend supplementing 10 to 15mg of zinc every day as well as eating a zinc rich diet.

14

Can Copper Cause Arthritis?

Copper is an essential mineral for the body. It is involved in the anti-oxidant enzyme SOD and reduces inflammation in the joints. It also helps to make red blood cells and the insulating layer around nerves. However copper can also be toxic if you get too much as the story of a patient of mine illustrates.

Mrs M's osteoarthritis had been getting continually worse over the past five years. No conventional treatment had helped ease the pain in her joints and even changing her diet and taking vitamin supplements had done little for her. I asked her if anything improved her condition. She said that she only felt better when she stayed at a friend's cottage in the country. She had once tried a copper bracelet, but that had made her worse. A hair mineral analysis revealed copper levels three times higher than the normal level. The most common source of excess copper is from copper water pipes. If the plumbing is new, or the water is soft, significant amounts of copper leach into water. Mrs M drank plenty of water from the tap, except when she stayed at her friend's cottage where the water came from a spring. Could it be that she was being poisoned by too much copper in her water?

The problem with excess copper is that it competes with zinc. Both are needed to fight inflammation. However, too much copper and not enough zinc could make inflammation worse, not better. Drinking large quantities of water passing through copper pipes can give you more than enough, especially if the water in your area is soft, which leaches more copper, and the plumbing is new, which means the pipes and joints have yet to be calcified.

On average, we need at least ten times as much zinc as copper. If your intake of copper comes from whole foods, including nuts, seeds, lentils, beans and fruits this is fine because they also contain zinc. However, if your diet does not include such foods, and you drink unfiltered water that passes through copper pipes you could accumulate too much. Taking the birth control pill also increases the retention of copper.

The Benefits of Copper

Copper levels in the blood and joints of arthritics are often very high. One study found three times as much copper in the synovial fluid of rheumatoid arthritics[33]. Rather than being a sign of toxicity, these high copper levels are thought to occur precisely because the body is fighting inflammation. Zinc and iron levels are also often raised. When arthritics go into remission copper levels fall[34]. However, during active arthritis, stores of copper in the liver fall. This suggests that, unless already overloaded with copper, the requirement for copper is greater in an arthritis sufferer. Many studies have also shown greater benefit from supplementing copper salicylate, rather than just salicylic acid (aspirin), suggesting again that copper has an important anti-inflammatory effect [35].

This may explain why some people benefit from copper bracelets. The benefit of copper bracelets was put to the test in one study where 240 arthritic patients were given either a copper bracelet or a 'placebo' bracelet to wear for a month[36]. After a month those with the copper bracelet were given a placebo bracelet and vice versa. of those who noted a difference in their condition between month one and month two significantly more improved when wearing the copper bracelet. Those who had previously worn a copper bracelet, and then wore the placebo bracelet got worse.

So, copper can help some and hinder others depending on your current copper status. I recommend a hair mineral analysis or an equivalent test for any arthritis sufferer. A hair mineral analysis also gives useful information about other minerals.

15

Calcium, Magnesium & Vitamin D - The Right Balance

Calcium is the most abundant mineral in the body, accounting for 1.6% of our body mass. Of the 1,200 grams of calcium in us more than 99% is found in the bones and teeth. The rest is present in muscles, nerves and the blood stream where it plays a crucial role in many enzymes and the production of nerve signals and muscular energy.

Calcium is relatively well absorbed, with on average 30% of ingested calcium reaching the blood-stream. But its absorption into the blood-stream depends on many factors. An excess of alcohol, a lack of hydrochloric acid, or an excess of acid forming foods (mainly protein) decrease its absorption. So does the presence of lead and other toxic minerals which competes for absorption sites. A hormone produced by the parathyroid gland also helps absorb calcium. It does this by converting vitamin D into another hormone which makes the gut wall more permeable to calcium. So lack of vitamin D is another factor to consider. Parathormone also helps to keep calcium in circulation once absorbed, by reducing excretion of calcium via the kidneys.

Once in the body, there are many factors which influence calcium balance. Once again, heavy metals like lead compete with calcium. So does sodium, tea, cocoa and red wine. In post-menopausal women the low levels of oestrogen also make calcium less retainable. One of the greatest factors is exercise or rather, lack of it. Studies by NASA, who had discovered losses of calcium in astronauts in zero gravity, shows that weight bearing exercise, for example walking, has the ability to raise calcium levels in the body by 2% or more 37.

Once in the body calcium is constantly moving from blood to

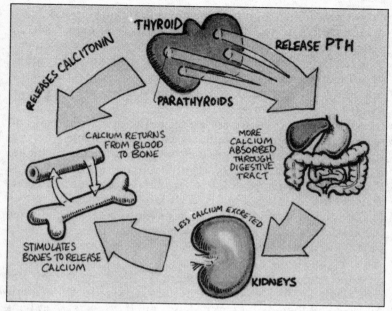

Figure 16 Calcium Balance

bone. The release of calcium into the blood occurs when it is needed to stimulate muscles or nerves. Once this reaction is over the thyroid gland recalls calcium to the bones by secreting the hormone calcitonin. An imbalance in the thyroid or parathyroid gland can also interfere with calcium balance.

Bones contain magnesium and phosphorus, as well as calcium. While phosphorus is abundant in most people's diets, calcium and magnesium are often deficient. Dairy produce, although a good source of calcium, is not a good source of magnesium. Nuts, seeds and root vegetables are good sources of both. Since most people's diet contains dairy produce, but little in the way of vegetables, nuts and seeds, magnesium is commonly deficient. Rough estimates predict that less than 20 per cent of people get enough magnesium[38].

The Importance of Magnesium

Without magnesium, calcium is unlikely to be used properly. Recent research has shown that magnesium deficient infants cannot produce enough parathormone (PTH) to respond to low calcium levels in the blood, consequently resulting in calcium deficiency in the body[39]. What's more the conversion of vitamin D into the active hormone that increases calcium retention is dependent on magnesium[40]. In order to be incorporated into bone, calcium forms crystals. The enzyme responsible for this is magnesium dependent [41].

Low magnesium levels are associated with osteoporosis and research by Dr Guy Abraham has shown remarkable results in reversing osteoporosis using a multi-nutrient approach including magnesium [40]. He studied 26 post-menopausal women all receiving hormone replacement therapy. All women were assessed for bone density. Seven patients received dietary advice similar to that recommended in this book, while nineteen received the same dietary advice and 6 nutritional supplements. These provided a broad spectrum of vitamins and minerals, including 500mg of calcium and 600mg of magnesium.

At their return visits, 6 to 12 months later, bone density was measured again. Those with dietary advise and hormone replacement therapy had an insignificant 0.7% increase in bone density, while those also taking supplements had a sixteen times greater increase in bone density of 11%. At the start of the study 15 out of the 19 women due to take supplements had a bone density below the fracture threshold indicating osteoporosis. Within a year of taking supplements only 7 patients still had bone densities below this threshold. This study shows, without a doubt, how potent a combined intake of vitamins and minerals is for reversing bone disease, in comparison to standard drug treatment.

Magnesium is also important in an increasingly common problem called *polymyalgia*. This describes a condition in which muscles throughout the body become stiff and painful. This condition is increasingly common, particularly among older women. One theory is that it is due to a defect in energy production within muscle cells, leading to build-up of the wrong chemicals, causing muscle pain and stiffness. Magnesium malate, which is magnesium plus malic acid, both of which are needed for proper energy production, has been shown in pilot trials to produce good results. This new approach, however, is not yet proven.

Vitamin D - The Sunlight Vitamin

Vitamin D is also needed to help calcium to be used properly by the body. It is converted into a hormone, calcitriol, that works with parathormone to absorb and retain calcium.

Vitamin D can be made in the skin in the presence of sunlight which may be one reason why arthritis sufferers often feel better in the summer. It is also present in meat, fish, eggs and milk. Some meat eaters get too much vitamin D from eating these foods, plus foods fortified with vitamin D. However, if you don't eat these foods often it is best to supplement 400ius of vitamin D each day. While supplementing vitamin D on its own is not effective for increasing bone density in osteoporosis it is effective together with calcium and other nutrients [42]. Supplementing the active hormone, calcitriol is the most effective of all [43]. This suggests that those with osteoporosis, and perhaps arthritis, have difficulty converting vitamin D into the active hormone calcitriol. Magnesium deficiency is one factor that could help this conversion to take place.

In summary, the body can use calcium better, helping to make strong bones and joints, if your diet also provides adequate amounts of magnesium and vitamin D. Supplementing an extra 500mg of calcium and magnesium, plus 400ius of vitamin D is likely to offer optimal protection for bones and joints. Another little known mineral that strengthens the bones is boron, the subject of the next chapter.

16

Boron for Healthy Bones

Boron is an abundant trace element in soil, food and in man. Most people consume about 3mg a day, mainly from vegetables[44]. High levels tend to be found in apples, pears, tomatoes, soya, prunes, raisins, dates and honey. Boron is an essential element for plants possibly affecting the control of plant growth hormones.

Although it has not yet been proven essential in man boron is found in the human body. It appears to be more concentrated in the thyroid and parathyroid glands which may suggest a role in their function. Animal studies point to an interaction between boron and calcium balance. Deficiency of vitamin D increases the need for boron and it is suspected that boron is somehow involved with the action of the parathyroid hormone, which helps maintain calcium within bone. Animals given boron supplements were found to be much less susceptible to the effects of magnesium deficiency. In plants boron is involved with the transport of calcium. According to Professor Derek Bryce-Smith "It would be surprising if such effects were confined to the animal kingdom" [45].

Boron and Arthritis

Although only one properly controlled double-blind trial has been published, there have been many reports linking boron with arthritis. Dr Newnham, working in New Zealand reported the successful treatment of rheumatoid arthritis with low doses of boron [46]. He noted that areas with low levels of boron in the soil, such as Mauritius and Jamaica, had high incidences of arthritis, while areas with high boron soil levels, such as Israel, have a very low incidence of arthritis. He reported that supplementing 6 to 9mg of boron per day improved symptoms within a few weeks in 80 to 90% of cases. He has also shown that boron supplementation can completely cure arthritis in horses, cattle, and dogs. In support of this concept, Dr Neil Ward from the University of Surrey, found lower levels of boron in the bones of rheumatoid arthritics compared to those without arthritis [47].

Dr Neilson and colleagues from the US Department of Agriculture investigated boron in relation to mineral and hormone balance in postmenopausal women [48]. They found that supplementing 3mg a day helped the body to retain calcium and magnesium, especially in those with poor magnesium status. It also increased the levels of the hormones testosterone and oestradiol, related to oestrogen, whiich is the only agent so far tested that consistently increases bone density in post-menopausal women. According to Dr Neilson "The findings suggest that supplementation of a low-level diet with an amount of boron commonly found in diets high in fruits and vegetables induces changes in postmenopausal women consistent with the prevention of calcium loss and bone demineralisation."

In 1990 the first double-blind trial on boron and arthritis was conducted [49]. Ten arthritic patients were placed on boron (6mg) and ten on placebo pills. Of the ten on boron five improved, while only one improved on placebo. There were no side-effects.

According to Professor Derek Bryce-Smith from the University of Reading, who has extensively researched the evidence about boron, "There is now a considerable body of evidence, much of good scientific quality, pointing to boron as an essential, or at least beneficial, factor in the metabolism of animals including humans. Osteoporosis and rheumatoid arthritis are the two diseases at present most probably associated with a low boron status. Although further scientific and medical studies in this area are needed, the evidence already available suggests that boron supplementation at a level of, say, 3mg per day, would be worth considering for both prophylaxis and treatment of diseases in men and postmenopausal women associated with structural disorders in bone of otherwise unknown aetiology (cause), and that this would carry little or no risk of adverse side-effects."

These early studies of boron used daily supplements of 3mg to 9mg of boron, given as sodium borate. Some supplements now combine calcium, or calcium and magnesium, with boron. Supplementing up to 3mg a day, together with a high fruit and vegetable diet, would provide optimal intakes of this probably important trace element.

17

Which Supplements Are Best?

Most of the elements essential for health are supplied from food to the body as a compound, bound to a larger (food) molecule. This binding is known as chelation, from the Greek word 'chela', a claw. Some form of chelation is important since most essential minerals in their 'raw' state are positively charged. The gut wall is negatively charged, so once separated from food through the process of digestion these unbound minerals would become loosely bound to the gut wall. Instead of being absorbed these minerals easily become bound to undesirable substances like phytic acid in bran, tannic acid in tea, oxalic acid and so on. These acids remove the mineral from the body.

Absorption of minerals is aided by attaching the mineral to an amino acid, or protein constituent. The amino acid containing the mineral is then more readily absorbed. Such forms of minerals are called 'amino acid chelated'. (They are also termed an 'organic' compound which is a definition of chemistry and has nothing to do with organic farming.) Examples of amino acid chelates are methionates, aspartates and picolinates. Some so-called amino acid chelates are better than others. This depends on how well bound the mineral is to the amino acid. If it is loosely bound it may separate during digestion. There is a patented process called the Albion process that guarantees a high quality chelate, and is used by some companies.

The best form of chelate depends mainly on how the body makes use of the mineral. For example, the iron in meat is in a chelated form the body can use directly for making haemoglobin, a constituent of red blood cells. It is probable, for example, that the superior results achieved with chromium picolinate are due to it being in a more similar form to that which the body uses than other forms of chromium.

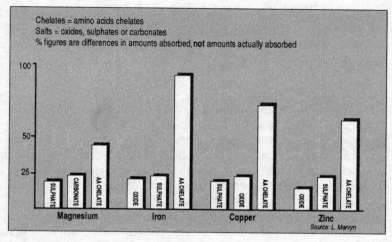

Chelates = amino acids chelates
Salts = oxides, sulphates or carbonates
% figures are differences in amounts absorbed, **not** amounts actually absorbed

Source: L. Mervyn

Figure 17 Comparative Absorption of Different Mineral Compounds

For some minerals the extra cost of amino acid chelated minerals outweighs the advantage. For example, calcium amino acid chelate is only twice as well absorbed as calcium carbonate, an inexpensive source of calcium. Iron amino acid chelate, on the other hand, is fout times as well absorbed as ferrous oxide making the price differential worth it. Generally speaking, the following forms are most available to the body, listed in order of their bio-availability.

Calcium & magnesium - *amino acid chelate, gluconate, citrate, carbonate*
Iron - *amino acid chelate, gluconate*
Zinc - *picolinate, amino acid chelate, citrate, gluconate*
Chromium - *picolinate, amino acid chelate, gluconate*
Selenium - *cysteine or methionine compound, amino acid chelate, gluconate*
Manganese - *amino acid chelate, gluconate*

As far as vitamins are concerned there is less variation from type to type. Vitamin C can be taken as ascorbic acid or calcium ascorbate, the latter being less acidic. Large amounts of calcium ascorbate should not be taken at meal times since this may reduce the level of acid in the stomach and negatively affect digestion.

Both forms are well tolerated. Dr Linus Pauling and Dr Cathcart recommend taking up to the 'bowel tolerance level'. This is the level below that which induces loose bowels. This may be anywhere between 1 and 15 grams a day. I recommend you start with a more modest dose of 3 grams.

The natural form of vitamin E is called d-alpha tocopherol (or tocopheryl) which is 30% more potent than the synthetic dl-alpha tocopherol. The natural form is preferable.

Vitamin B3 is best in the non-blushing niacinamide form, and B5 as calcium pantothenate. Vitamin B6 (pyridoxine) has to be converted into the active form known as pyridoxal-5-phosphate (P5P) before it can be used by the body. The enzyme that does this is zinc dependent. For best utilisation of vitamin B6 either take pyridoxal-5-phosphate, or take vitamin B6 with zinc. Supplements are available which contain, for example, 100mg of vitamin B6 and 10mg of zinc.

Part 4

The Right Exercises & The Right Attitude

18

Going Straight

A good way of viewing health is to consider that we have three domains: physical, chemical and psychological. If all three are in balance disease is unlikely to occur. Nutrition is all about bringing the body's chemistry back into balance. This chapter and Chapter 20, Anti-Arthritis Exercises, are all about the physical side of arthritis.

Physical imbalance or strain will ultimately cause joint damage however good your nutrition is. So there is little point improving your nutrition if you make no changes to underlying causes of mechanical stress. In practical terms this means two things: identifying mechanical stresses and imbalances; and correcting them and the behaviour that caused them to develop.

The Causes of Joint Strain

Joint strain usually occurs for one or more of the following reasons. The first is one-off traumas or accidents. These may occur any time in life, including childhood. A bad fall, a sports related injury, a car accident or any other trauma can throw out the body's mechanics so that the musculature has to adapt a new posture to compensate. But it cannot compensate for ever, and the result may be joint strain, leading to arthritis.

The result can occur from small amounts of trauma over a long period of time. This may be repetitive strain inducing actions in your occupation or sporting activities, for example, repetitive lifting of things in the wrong way, or typing in the wrong position.

Then there are long-term postural factors to consider such as how you sit, lie down, walk and move around. These too can induce strain over long periods of time.

In fact, our posture and way of moving is the result of everything that has happened to us up until now, including injuries, accidents and occupations long forgotten. The body, however, never forgets.

The first sign of mechanical imbalances is periodic pain - the odd back pain or joint pain. This is well worth paying attention to since it is the body registering discomfort. Pain itself can be seen as the body's way of protecting an area, in this case by encouraging you to inhibit movement. In this light arthritis could be seen as the body's way of immobilising joints that can no longer take any more strain.

The skeleton of the body is much more than a mechanical structure. It is a storehouse of minerals, a factory for new cells and a protected conduit for nerves and blood vessels. From each spinal vertebra extends a nerve, vein and artery. If the spine is compressed this will affect both the blood supply and nerve supply, not only to the spine itself, but also to other parts of the body, under control of these vital nerve signals. Changes in the structure of the body will affect its function. That is why a wide variety of heath problems can be the result of musculo-skeletal imbalances.

Identifying and Correcting Mechanical Imbalances

Identifying and correcting mechanical imbalances is the purpose of osteopathy, chiropractic and physiotherapy and is an essential part of the proper treatment of all musculo-skeletal diseases including arthritis. These practitioners can identify what the problem is by palpation, by measuring and analysing how you move, and sometimes by X-ray. Palpation involves feeling not only the position and mobility of joints but the nature of the soft tissue which includes ligaments, tendons and muscle. An experienced practitioner learns much from palpation. The goal of these therapies is to increase your flexibility and ability to adapt to different physical demands so that you can go about your life with the least strain. (See Useful Addresses on page 158 to find your nearest practitioner.)

By working on soft tissue with massage techniques, and on bone alignment though manipulation, corrections to joint structure can be made. These must be backed up with exercise or corrections to mechanical behaviour to maintain and improve mechanical function. By improving movement within a joint the blood supply and nerve function may also improve helping the joint to heal faster.

While osteopaths, chiropractors and physiotherapists can point you in the right direction your mechanical health depends mainly on what you do. The first step is increased awareness of your body as a complex and incredible instrument. With awareness you may begin to notice how you put your body into stress. If you have weak or tense areas you may benefit greatly from regular massage, regular check-ups and specific exercises. Mechanical health depends on regular exercise to maintain flexibility and strength. This is a vital part of your anti-arthritis programme and is covered in Chapter 20.

There are many other excellent exercises and techniques that help re-educate you and your body. These include the Alexander technique, Feldenkrais, postural integration, hatha yoga and others and are highly recommended. In the Alexander Technique, rather than correcting mechanical imbalances in the body itself, the focus is on correcting the behaviour that led to that imbalance. Habitual ways of reacting physically, can, when repeated over many years lead to joint trauma. This, in turn can lead to arthritis. By identifying the particular pattern of movement that is traumatising the body, and changing that pattern of movement the joints and muscles have a chance to heal. Such re-education techniques are probably most applicable in osteoarthritis and arthritis which stems from a physical trauma. Useful addresses are given at the back of the book.

The Importance of Sitting Correctly

Two critical activities that we spend a lot of time doing are sitting and lying down. How you sit can make unnecessary demands on your muscles and ligaments, restrict your breathing and impair your circulation.

Most office chairs are not designed for good sitting. However, there are some simple adjustments you can make to your sitting environment and how you sit to reduce unnecessary stress. First of all, the chair you sit on needs to be the right height for your work surface so that you don't have to slouch and collapse your spine and chest to do your work. You may need to increase the height or lower it. Since it is good to have your feet firmly on the floor, if you are short you may work best by putting something firm on the ground, like a couple of telephone directories, to rest your feet on.

When you sit make sure you sit straight on the sitting bones which are the curved ridges of bone that you can feel at the base of the pelvis when sitting. If you sit on the sitting bones your spine has more chance of being straight. Often we slouch back, collapsing the spine and resting on the coccyx.

Now check your eye position. If you get eye strain you may well be getting joint and spine strain too. The eyes literally lead the nervous system. You will automatically adjust your body to see whatever you are working on. If you are too high you will strain forward. Experiment with changing the angle and height of material you are reading or, if you use a computer, the level of the screen in relation to you. if you are typing material alter the angle of the material you read so that it is easiest to read. Angled writing surfaces, like old school desks, and angled copy holders, like lecterns, help to reduce unnecessary strain.

Your arms also need to be in the correct position. Armchairs can encourage you to lift your shoulders to rest your arms on the arms

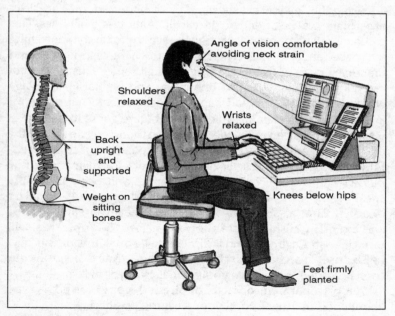

Figure 18 Correct Sitting Position

of the chairs. This creates unnecessary strain. Your shoulders should be down and back at all times. Check that your arms, elbows and wrists can remain flexible while you work so there is neither strain nor restricted circulation. Rest your hands in your lap when you are not working.

If you do spend a lot of time at a desk I recommend an excellent book by Julie Friedberger called Office Yoga (see recommended reading on page 151). This book gives simple exercises that you can do to improve flexibility. These exercises are good for anyone with arthritis.

The Dangers of Going To Bed

We spend up to a third of our lives lying down. How you lie makes all the difference to your musculo-skeletal system for two reasons. The first is because bad sleeping positions or conditions, such as too soft a mattress, introduce strain to the body. The second is that the spine and other joints are nourished when you lie down.

During the day you get shorter. Between the vertebrae are discs of cartilage that is softer than the cartilage at the end of bones. This cartilage gets compressed through the action of gravity, shortening the space between discs. When you lie down the discs expand and literally suck in nutrients from adjoining tissues. This method of receiving nutrients is called imbibition and is vital for cartilage which has no direct blood supply. You can help nourish your joints by doing loosening up exercises before going to bed.

Most people sleep in the foetal position, lying on one side or the other, with legs flexed. This is fine provided the surface is correct. Either too soft a mattress, too hard a mattress, too many or too few pillows can introduce strain to the spine and neck. Generally speaking the spine should be horizontal and not unduly flexed up or down. Thus a soft mattress that forces the lower spine to sink, and too many cushions that allow the neck to flex upwards, will introduce strain. If you find it difficult to lie on your side this may be because of mechanical imbalances. It is also fine to sleep on your back provided the surface you lie on is firm enough.

Your osteopath, chiropractor or physiotherapist can advise you about good mattresses and your sleeping position.

19

Hydrotherapy

Water is the most important nutrient for the human body. Your body is 65% water. While you can survive for a month without food, go a few days without water and death will ensue. Water, which is hydrogen and oxygen ($H2O$), has remarkable properties. It can store, absorb and transmit heat very effectively as ice, water or steam. It is remarkably non-toxic and therefore can be used internally and externally. (There is a case of a man dying after drinking 3 litres of water in 20 minutes. This shows that almost everything is toxic dependent on the dose.) It has been used therapeutically for thousands of years by cultures all over the world. In India, for example, the Rig Veda, thought to be written about 1,500 BC, states that "water cures the fever's glow". Hippocrates used water treatments extensively aroud 400 BC he writes "for the bath soothes pain in the side, chest and back; cuts the sputum, promotes expectoration, improves the respiration, and allays lassitude; for it soothes the joints and outer skin."

Hydrotherapy means the use of water in any form for the maintenance of health or the treatment of disease. At different times in history hydrotherapy has been popular. It is a very popular naturopathic technique in Germany, but not so known in Britain. Dr Kellogg, writing in the 1900's in America, was a great advocate of hydrotherapy. Differing opinions still exist about its importance. A major review article in 1983 concluded that its positive effects were limited to external effects, helping to reduce pain but not changing the underlying basis of disease. Yet an article in a German medical journal reported that after hydrotherapy there were increased concentrations of immune complexes not seen in control patients not receiving hydrotherapy [1].

Hydrotherapy and Arthritis

Whether or not hydrotherapy can improve immune function it is a very useful and safe method for reducing localised pain, inflammation and improving circulation. Exposing an inflamed area to cold water has a depressant, calming effect and may be a useful way of calming down inflamed joints. However, if the temperature is too cold, for example the use of ice compresses, there is a reaction which is stimulating rather than calming, and not desirable for an actively inflamed and hot area.

On the other hand, stimulation of circulation to a joint is generally beneficial, helping to remove toxins and improve the supply of nutrients to the joints, as well as stimulating the movement of fluid within joints, needed to nourish the cartilage. Improving circulation to a joint is best achieved with alternating hot and cold, usually in the form of compresses.

Compresses

Two simple procedures may be helpful in your anti-arthritis strategy. The first is the cold compress. This is used to calm down joints that are actively inflamed and hot. If you are slightly feverish as well this is a good indication that a cold compress is suitable. Put cold water and ice into a bowl of water, or basin. The temperature on the water should be between 13 and 18°C (55 and 65°F) which should feel cold but not result in pain or numbness. Soak a towel in this water, wring it out, and place it on the affected area. You will need to soak and ring out the towel every 2 or 3 minutes to maintain the cold temperature. Do this for about 10 minutes then dry the area. The cold compress is reported to reduce pain and inflammation. This may be particularly useful in rheumatoid arthritis, gout, bursitis, tendonitis, and tenosynovitis. If the water is much too cold the body can react to the extreme cold and heat up the joint instead. So be careful to get the temperature right. You'll soon find out what works for you.

The alternating hot and cold compress is used to improve circulation to a joint or area of the body that has become congested. Often, arthritic joints have little movement and poor circulation. Heat improves circulation and flexibility. So too does extreme cold by causing a heating reaction. This combination may help to get nutrients to the joints, and toxic material away and has been shown to increase blood flow to extremities by 95% [1]. There are differing views about the length of each phase. I recommend you try a hot compress for 3 minutes, followed by a cold compress for 30 to 60 seconds, and repeat this 3 times. Make a bowl of hot water (around 37 to 40°C or 98 to 104°F) hot enough to produced skin redness if prolonged but not so hot that have to take your hand out. Soak a towel in this, and wring out then apply to the affected area. Soak another towel in cold water, wring out and wrap around ice cubes which will help to keep the towel very cold. Apply this after 3 minutes for 30 to 60 seconds. Ice packs can also be used for the cold compress.

Therapeutic Baths

Another useful way of stimulating circulation is to have a cold shower after a hot bath or shower. If you are trying to stimulate circulation in a particular area then shower this area with cold just for enough time to cool the area down. Your body will respond by warming it up, leaving you with a healthy glow after the shower. This would be particularly good to do before an exercise session as part of your warm up.

After an exercise session you may benefit from a bath containing sodium bicarbonate. This alkalises the water and the skin and is reputed to help the body detoxify. After therapeutic massage, or exercise there can be more acid end-products of metabolism. Drinking a glass of water containing sodium bicarbonate (such as Eno's) and having a warm bath with 100g of sodium bicarbonate in it is thought to help reduce stiffness. Sodium bicarbonate is the same thing as bicarbonate of soda, used to bake cakes. A 100g tub can be bought for less than 40 pence. Enos can be bought in sachets to drink with water. Take this after an exercise session or therapeutic massage.

A few words of caution: check the water temperature with a thermometer the first time you try these compresses. Do not use the hot/cold compress if you are diabetic without your doctor or naturopath's permission. Naturopaths are fully trained in hydrotherapy techniques, many of which are more advanced than those I have described. Should you wish to explore this avenue further I recommend you consult a naturopath .

Water Exercises

As well as its heating and cooling effects water provides resistance to the body which, in itself improves the flow of fluid within joints. Water pressure, for example, showers or jacuzzis are particularly good for this. Water also provides extra resistance which makes it the ideal medium for exercising in without straining the joints. Many of the exercises referred to in Chapter 28 can be done in water. Some can be done in the bath. I recommend at least one session a week of exercise in water for any kind of arthritic condition.

20
Anti-Arthritis Exercises

Exercise is an important part of an anti-arthritis programme. Through exercise joints are nourished and prevented from seizing up. Cartilage, since it does not have a blood supply, relies on movement of the joint to supply nutrients. Resistance exercise also increases bone density, helping to prevent osteoporosis. Weightlessness studies at NASA have found that, in the absence of gravity, bones start to degenerate. Just walking around exercises muscles. Bone density increases with weight bearing exercise - unless you are a bear. Research has shown that the bones of hibernating bears actually become more dense. It appears that, unlike us, a sleeping bear recycles its own calcium, rather than losing it.

The effects of exercise on bone mineral content were compared with the the effects of supplementing 750mg of calcium and 400ius of vitamin D over a three year period. The elderly women on this trial did 30 minutes of mild physical exercises while sitting in a chair, three times a week. At the end of the trial their bone mineral content had increased 2.29%, while those on supplements alone had increased 1.58%. Those doing no exercise, nor taking supplements had a decrease in bone mineral content of 3.29%. This study illustrates just how important exercise is for bone strength[2].

Exercise also boosts the immune system. T'ai Chi was shown to increase T-cell count (needed for immunity) by 40%. However, overtraining or vigorous exercise can actually depress immune function[3].

Strength, Suppleness and Stamina

There are three important aspects to exercise - strength, suppleness and stamina. We need strength to function and give support to the body. Strengthening exercises also help to increase bone density. Suppleness of muscles and joints declines with age, unless you exercise to keep yourself supple. Naturally, the joints you exercise the least become less supple. Your muscles may be compensating for bad posture, paving the way for problem areas later in life. Appropriate exercise can develops stamina by making demands on the heart and cardiovascular system to supply oxygen and nutrients to the working muscles. Increased stamina means decreased risk for cardiovascular disease.

Different kinds of exercise involve different amounts of these three key factors. Yoga is excellent for suppleness. Brisk walking is good for stamina. Gardening and physical hobbies are often good for strength. Swimming, on the other hand, is good for all three.

The Benefits of Exercise

In case you think that eating the right diet is enough, consider this study by Bill Solomon from the University of Arizona, who decided to find out which was more important for health - diet or exercise [4]. He got some obliging pigs to run around a track but fed them the average vitamin-deficient diet. Another group had the pig-equivalent of health food but had no exercise. A third group of pigs both exercised and ate a healthy diet. The third group did best overall, proving that both exercise and diet are most beneficial to health.

Regular exercise has many potential benefits in relation to arthritis. It supplies nutrients to the joints, lubricates and nourishes them, strengthens bones, increases mobility and decreases pain and stiffness, relaxes muscles, and reduces joint strain by keeping your weight down. On top of all that it keeps your heart, arteries and lungs healthy, improves energy and sleep.

Exercise for Arthritis - The Golden Rules

It is, however, very important not to over-exercise or wrongly exercise affected joints. Take great care not to overstress arthritic joints. It is neither necessary to feel pain for exercise to do you good, nor is it advisable. Of course, sometimes there is a degree of pain, especially after exercising muscles that have been inactive. A good guideline is that if you experience pain induced by exercise for more than two hours after the exercise you are working too hard. Do a little less next time.

Protect yourself from unneccessary strain from certain exercises. For example, if you like walking or jogging, get a really supportive pair of shoes and walk on grass rather than on the road. Rebounders are a great way of reducing strain on the knees and hips. Exercise done in water is the best of all. Many anti-arthritis exercises can be done either in the bath or in a swimming pool.

Osteoarthritis benefits most from regular exercise that is both strengthening and increases flexibility in affected joints. Improved strength supports the joint, while flexibility discourages the formation of spurs. Both nourish the joint by increasing circulation of fluid.

Rheumatoid arthritis requires care. Rheumatic joints require periods of rest and periods of exercise. Over-exercising can cause flare-ups which are to be avoided. If joints are actively inflamed, hot and painful they should not be vigourously exercised although they can be passively taken through their range of movement at different times during the day. Yoga exercises are particularly good here.

However, because of periods of relative inactivity, when your joints aren't inflamed its important to exercise them and develop some strength.

Your Exercise Programme

Think of exercise as one of the natural remedies you are employing to cure your arthritis. No doubt you will follow a diet and take supplements virtually every day. The same thing applies to exercise. You need to establish a routine and stick to it.

At minimum, aim for 15 minutes exercise each day. This may increase to 30 minutes. Two days a week it may be swimming, one day a week it may be a walk, leaving three days a week to do a routine at home.

Pick a time in the day, preferably when you feel good, not exhausted. Make sure you will not be disturbed so you can have 15 to 30 minutes of peace, simply exercising. This itself is calming. Joints and muscles benefit most from exercise once they have been stretched and 'warmed up'. Simple exercises that take joints through their range of movement is a good way to warm up before doing more demanding exercises. You may wish to start by focussing specifically on one problem area. This is quite useful in that you can soon get a sense of what effect regular exercise has on a set of joints. Ultimately it is better, however, to exercise the whole body. End your exercise session with some simple stretches, much like the warm up. This helps to maintain the flexibility you have created while exercising. After exercising is a great time to take a bath or apply one of the hydrotherapy techniques discussed in the last chapter.

Setting Goals and Sticking to Them

Once you've worked out what you need to do to maintain suppleness, strength and stamina now you need to stick to it! It is always essential to plan your routine, write it down and monitor your progress. Draw up a routine, Monday to Sunday, that you can follow. Don't be over-ambitious. Honestly ask yourself if what you have set is realistic and achievable. It is much better to succeed at a low-level programme than fail and ditch exercise all together. When you've worked out a viable and effective programme display this somewhere you can see it every day.

If you go off your programme, perhaps missing exercise for a few days when other events take over, remember to get back to the programme. I remind myself at the beginning of each week to follow my routine. Whatever I did yesterday or last week becomes irrelevant. What is relevant is doing my routine scheduled for today. The guidelines in Chapter 29 will help you monitor your progress and keep yourself motivated.

21

The Psychosomatic Side of Arthritis

The word psychosomatic is not an insult, as some would believe. It literally means mind-body and is used to describe connections between one's mental and emotional state and physical state. There is little question that arthritis, particularly rheumatoid arthritis, can create major life stresses both for the sufferer and their family [5]. But, to what extent does psychological state cause or encourage physical changes that lead to arthritis?

As long ago as 1936 the onset of rheumatoid arthritis was associated with major stress such as marital pressures, work-related stress and worry [6]. More recent controlled studies have confirmed that those who develop rheumatoid arthritis often have difficulty adjusting to difficult life experiences [7].

Research at the Arthritis and Rheumatism Foundation and at the University of Southern California Medical School has shown a link between arthritis and emotional stress [8]. "Hidden anger, fear or worry often accompanies the beginning of arthritis" says Dr Austin from the University of Southern California, who believes that many arthritics have difficulty expressing anger and may turn it in on themselves.

Dr Ronald Lamont-Havers, while national medical director of the Arthritis and Rheumatism Foundation, examined hundreds of prison inmates and found only a negligible incidence of RA. he told the Los Angeles Times why: "These individuals who let out their angers and aggressive feelings so violenty that they wound up behind bars had practically no RA. Emotional stress, brought on by hidden anger, fear or worry, often accompanies the beginning of arthritis." [9]

Many ancient philosophies and modern psychologies consider the mind and body to be intimately connected. Imbalances in a particular system in the body are thought to correspond with mental and emotional imbalances that may seek expression through the physical body. According to Oscar Ichazo, who developed the Arica system, the musculo-skeletal system is the physical manifestation of a person's need for space, authority and ownership. According to this theory a person who has been denied their own space and authority throughout childhood and adult life may be more prone to developing musculo-skeletal problems.

The psychologist Louise Hay believes "we create every so-called 'illness' in our body. The body, like everything else in life, is a mirror of our inner thoughts and beliefs. It is always talking to us, if we only take time to listen." In her book, *You Can Heal Your Life*,[10] she makes the following observations in relation of arthritic-type problems: "Arthritis is a disease that comes from a constant pattern of criticism. First of all, criticism of the self, and then criticism of other people. Arthritic people attract a lot of criticism because it is their pattern to criticize. They are cursed with 'perfectionism', the need to be perfect at all times in every situation." Through her work she has noticed a pattern of criticism, resentment and feeling unloved in many of her clients with arthritis. "Guilt" she says "looks for punishment, and punishment looks for pain." She is careful to point out that "Not every mental equivalent is 100% true for everyone. However, it does give us a point of reference to begin the search for the cause of disease."

Chronic arthritis is itself a great stress [11]. It is sadly no surprise that a large proportion of rheumatoid arthritics have been found to suffer from depression, have marital difficulties and low self-esteem. One key factor is the thought of having a disease of unknown outcome with no knowledge of a treatment that really works. This leads to 'learned helplessness', the belief that effective solutions are not available to control or eliminate either the disease or other life stresses. People who have this attitude of mind are less likely to adjust well to changes and stresses in life and are more likely to be depressed [12].

As you will have discovered from this book, unless you have already exhausted all the nutritional approaches to arthritis, there is much you can do to improve the outcome of any form of arthritis, without the risk of side-effects. In this day and age, with rapid access to information we must all become more responsible for, and more in control of our own health. The same is true for life in general. There are always ways of dealing with stresses and difficult situations. So much depends on the right attitude. Chapter 27 gives a few simple and practical tips for coping with life's stresses.

22

Light - The Forgotten Nutrient

Research into light is still in its infancy, however we do already know that light is an essential nutrient for both mind and body. We receive the effects of light in two ways: through the skin and through the eyes. Both stimulate glands in the body and affect hormone levels.

The whole chemistry of the body is designed around these stimulating effects of light. For example, the reason you wake up is that light, entering through the translucent portions of the skull, stimulates both the pineal and pituitary gland in the brain which leads to increased adrenalin levels to allow us to wake up full of energy. If, however, you sleep with thick curtains drawn to exclude all natural light, and wake to the sound of an alarm clock how can you expect your body and mind to function at their best?

The skin contains a layer of cells which contain melanin, a dark pigment. Melanin filters out solar radiation very effectively. Africans, who have very high melanin levels, filter out between 50 and 95% of solar radiation. This adaptation may have served two purposes: firstly it prevents the skin from the oxidative effects of radiation responsible for the high skin cancer rate in white skinned people living in hot countries; secondly it limits the amount of vitamin D made in the skin, probably in order to prevent toxicity.

The Sunshine Vitamin

John Ott, now a leading expert in the importance of light, noticed in his previous job as a time lapse photographer for Walt Disney, that flowers responded differently under different lighting conditions. One of his specialities was photographing flowers from bud to blossom. Yet, under certain lights flowers wouldn't flower or fertilise. He now believes that we benefit from a full spectrum of light wavelengths, supplied by the sun, but not by most artificial light.

He now believes that full spectrum light must enter the eye and advocates we all spend some time outdoors in direct light, without glasses or contact lenses, which obscure the beneficial effect. He noticed that his arthritis improved when he started to spend time outdoors without glasses. Immunologist Jennifer Meek is convinced that even as little as three minutes of light entering the eye stimulates the immune system, which is under attack in arthritis.

Probably the most important effect of light is that it converts two chemicals, ergosterol and 7-dehydrocholesterol, found in layers of the skin, into vitamin D. "People who do not get adequate sunlight will have reduced formation in the skin of vitamin D2 and D3, rendering them vitamin D deficient if they are also not absorbing adequate vitamin D in the diet" says Dr Stephen Davies [13], who identifies dark-skinned people living in northern climates as particularly at risk. Others at risk include elderly housebound people, people living in urban northerly regions, and immigrants who rarely expose their skin to sunlight. So, for example, an Indian, who has dark skin and remains covered up much of the time, and is vegan, eating no meat, eggs or dairy products, is at risk of vitamin D deficiency. This causes rickets (in children) and osteolamalcia (in adults), diseases in which the bones become maliable. Africans, no doubt due to their high melanin content, are most susceptible to rickets. Even if you get enough calcium, a lack of UV radiation does impair the body's utilisation of calcium significantly, as shown by Dr Wurtman studying people at the Chelsea Soldiers Home in Massachusetts, USA [14].

Vitamin D, whether from diet or from the effects of sunlight on the skin, is converted into calcitriol, an active hormone that works with parathormone, produced in the parathyroid gland, to control calcium balance in the body. The amount you need depends on the amount you produce in the skin. Vitamin D production is apparently at its highest in the autumn, perhaps as an evolutionary adaptation to store up for the months ahead.

If you are mainly vegetarian and don't eat foods rich in vitamin D (such as eggs and dairy produce), and do not get substantial exposure to sunlight, I would recommend supplementing your diet with 400ius of vitamin D daily. This level is found in many mutivitamins and also in some calcium and magnesium supplements. If you live abroad and are exposed to substantial amounts of sunlight be careful that you are not getting too much dietary vitamin D because an excess has a negative effect on calcium balance.

Light in the Darkness

Light entering through the eye stimulates the brain which in turn shuts off melatonin production in the pineal gland. Melatonin, which is only produced in the absence of light, is one brain chemical that makes you sleepy. It is currently being researched in relation to sleep problems, jet lag and depression.

A proportion of people suffering from depression have what is called a seasonly affected disorder, SAD. Dr Norman Rosenthal from the US National Institute of Health wondered whether this might be to do with the length of exposure to daylight [15]. As the days get shorter these people got more depressed. To test this theory he exposed volunteers to full-spectrum light equivalent to sunlight for up to three hours before dawn and after dusk. A control group had the same routine to follow but were exposed to dimmer lighting equivalent to domestic lighting. While the dim lights made no difference all 13 of the SAD patients improved, some dramatically. Most found that they could once again cope with life and function in their job, while before they often entered a state of severe depression in the winter months.

While I am unaware of any studies that have examined the effects of light on arthritis the beneficial effects of living in a sunnier climate have been reported by many arthritis sufferers. On the basis of the evidence above, especially if your arthritis and/or state of mind definitely get worse in the late winter and early spring, you may benefit from more direct exposure to full spectrum light. You can achieve this by: spending more time outside, without glasses or contact lenses; taking a holiday to a sunny climate during the winter; and fitting full spectrum lighting into the main rooms you live and work in. Addresses of suppliers are given on page 158.

Part 5

The Anti-Arthritis Action Plan

23
Detoxify Yourself

Many of the foods and drinks we eat contain substances that are either toxic to the body or create adverse effects such as an allergic reaction. This 10 Day Detox Diet is designed to remove any foods that could have a bad effect including the most common allergy provoking foods, substances that upset blood sugar balance and known toxins. This gives your body a break - a chance to detoxify, stop reacting allergically, and even out your blood sugar levels. This diet should not be carried out for longer than ten days without the supervision of a doctor or qualified nutritionist.

If you have a history of blood sugar problems or diabetes, or any other complicating disease do not attempt this 10 Day Detox Diet without the supervision of your doctor or a qualifed nutritionist. They may wish to modify this in view of your overall health. In any event I recommend you line up a suitably qualified health professional whom you can call on should the need arise.

It is quite possible that you may feel worse in the first three days of this diet. This happens for a minority of people and is usually a sign that your body is detoxifying or suffering a type of withdrawal effect from either a stimulant or an allergy provoking food that you have become 'addicted' to. Symptoms may include headaches, aching muscles and joints, tiredness, or slight nausea. If these persist for more than three days, and there is no sign of improvement, then I suggest you seek the advice of a suitably qualified health professional. By day 3, however, most people feel physically fitter and mentally sharper.

Instead of monitoring your symptoms every week, using the system described in Chapter 29, monitor your symptoms every day. If you notice a definite improvement in any of your symptoms over the ten days use this opportunity to identify whether you are allergic or intolerant to any of the foods you've been avoiding. This you can do by using the Pulse Test explained in Chapter 26 as you reintroduce foods one by one.

What to Avoid

The following foods are excluded from all days: All foods containing grains (wheat, oats, barley, rye and corn); all dairy produce (milk, yoghurt, butter, cream whether from cow, sheep or goat); all red meat (beef, pork, lamb) tomatoes, peppers, aubergines; oranges, grapefruit; peanuts; sugar; chocolate; food colourings or chemical additives.

The following drinks are excluded from all days: Coffee including decaffeinated coffee; tea; drinks with added sugar or additives; alcohol. If you smoke and would like to stop this is a great time to do it. In any event smoking should be avoided or reduced as much as you possibly can.

What to Increase

By now you're probably wondering what on earth you can eat. The answer is there is plenty to choose from including all fruits and vegetables (other than those specifed to avoid), rice, millet, buckwheat and quinoa, all lentils and beans, all soya produce including soya milk and tofu, chicken, turkey and fish, all nuts and seeds (except peanuts). Since you may not be familiar with many of these foods and how to use them to make delicious meals the following page contains a list of suggested menus with the recipes being given in the next chapter. Any recipes marked 'DETOX' in Chapter 24 are suitable during these days.

Here are some useful substitutes for the foods you're used to eating:

Milk   have soya milk instead
Cream   make cashew cream by blending cashew nuts with water
Pasta   have buckwheat pasta
Cereal have sugar-free rice crispies or millet flakes with fruit
Meat   have chicken, turkey, fish, tofu or quorn
Bread   have rice cakes
Coffee/Tea have Rooibosch (red bush tea), herb or fruit teas
Alcohol have Aqua Libra
Chocolate have a Sunflower bar
Snacks have fresh fruit, or small quantities of dried fruit and
            a few almonds or sunflower seeds

Most of all, fill yourself up with lots of fruit and vegetables, rice, beans and lentils. Half the world live off these foods alone. You should be able to do it for ten days!

It is important to drink plenty of water during this detoxifying diet. If your body is eliminating toxic material drinking water will dilute it, thereby giving the kidneys, which cleanse the blood, an easier task. Instead of tea and coffee choose from the wide variety of tasty alternatives available in any health food shop. My favourites include Blackcurrant Bracer, Red Zinger, Emperors Choice, Raspberry Rendezvous - the list is extensive. You can also make your own. For example, try fresh ginger and cinnamon by putting six large slices of ginger and a stick of cinnamon in a thermos half full with boiling water and leaving for fifteen minutes.

Fruit juice is fine as long as it is sugar free and you dilute it with water to reduce the overall sweetness. Cherry juice is particularly beneficial. In season you can make a delicious drink by blending the entire flesh of a watermelon, pips and all. The husk of the seeds crack and sink to the bottom leaving the white seed, full of nutrients, in the drink. Two pints of this is a meal in itself and thoroughly detoxifying. Vegetable juice is also excellent. Two thirds carrot juice and one third beetroot juice is my favourite. Carrot and apple juice is another good combination. You may need to dilute this a little as it is quite sweet.

Supplementary Benefit

Two vitamins help to speed up purification of the body. These are vitamin C and vitamin B3 in the form of niacin. Niacin is different from niacinamide, which is recommended later for increasing joint flexibility. The niacin form of vitamin B3 is a 'vasodilator'. This means that the tiny blood vessels, called capillaries, that deliver nutrients to cells and collect toxins, dilate or enlarge. This helps them to nourish and detoxify cells. Niacin is used to help eliminate drug residues in the body and has been proven highly effective in helping drug addicts to withdraw and poison victims to recover. It also lowers high blood cholesterol levels.

Niacin consequently causes a temporary 'blush'. Your body goes red, a bit like a mild sunburn, you may got hot and a little itchy. This usually takes up to 15 minutes to happen and lasts for up to 30 minutes and is neither harmful nor unusual. In fact, it is very beneficial and illustrates just how potent nutrients are. Experiment with taking 100mg each day on an empty stomach. If nothing happens take 200mg. (Make sure you buy niacin, not niacinamide.) Since you can get a little cold after a niacin blush this is a great time to have a hot bath. I recommend taking niacin first in the morning, before breakfast, or before you go to bed. Initially your joints may ache more during the blush, and then show improvement. The effects of niacin are very calming.

Vitamin C also helps the body to detoxify and I therefore recommend taking 3 grams (3 x 1,000mg tablets, one with each meal) a day during the Detox Diet, plus a good multivitamin. So that's one all-round multivitamin, three 1,000mg vitamin C and one100mg niacin (B3) tablet each day.

Take It Easy

During these ten days take it easy. Make sure you get enough sleep. Do not overstress, overwork or overexercise yourself. A moderate amount of exercise is still advisable. Stock up with the foods, drinks and supplements you need in advance. Any health food shop will have most of the specialist foods and drinks I've mentioned here.

The 10 Day Detox Diet

Here are a list of suggested menus to help you. Recipes are given in the next chapter. Any of these meals can be substituted. The key point is to stay off the 'avoid' foods and drinks, eat plenty of fruit and vegetables and drink plenty of water.

DAY 1 & 5
Breakfast: Get Up & Go
Lunch: Baked Potato, Crudites and Satay Sauce
Dinner: Sweet and Sour Tofu and Watercress Salad
Snacks: Fresh fruit

DAY 2 & 6

Breakfast: Apple Muesli
Lunch: Tofu and Avocado Dip
Dinner: Mushroom Pilaf and Spinach and Bean Salad
Snacks: Fresh Fruit

DAY 3 & 7

Breakfast: Get Up & Go
Lunch: Nutty Three Bean Salad
Dinner: Chestnut Hotpot and Green Salad
Snacks: Fresh fruit

DAY 4 & 8

Breakfast: Fruity Millet Flakes
Lunch: Carrot Soup in the Raw
Dinner: Rice and Bean Casserole
Snacks: Fresh fruit

DAY 5 & 9

Breakfast: Get Up & Go
Lunch: Rice and Beansprout Salad
Dinner: Shepherdess Pie and Garden Salad
Snacks: Fresh fruit

DAY 6 & 10

Breakfast: Sesame Porridge
Lunch: Butter Bean and Sweetcorn Soup
Dinner: Buckwheat Spaghetti Napolitana and Green Salad
Snacks: Fresh fruit

24
The Anti-Arthritis Diet

The principles of eating to avoid arthritis are the same as those for overall good health. From the previous chapter, and the following chapter, you may have identified specific foods or food groups that make your symptoms worse. Obviously, these foods should be avoided. Even if no apparent reactions occurred I recommend limiting your intake of wheat products, especially baked wheat products such as bread, cakes and pastries, and dairy products, especially high fat foods such as cheese and cream. The basic guidelines are as follows:

DECREASE	INCREASE
Sugar	Vegetables
Tea and coffee	Fruit and berries
Alcohol	Seeds and nuts
Chocolate	Lentils, beans and peas
High fat meats	Quinoa and millet
Wheat products	Rice and rice cakes
Dairy products	Oats and oat cakes
	100% rye bread
	Soya products such as tofu
	Fish
	Fruit and herb teas
	Water and diluted fruit juice

Given that humanity has spent most of its life roaming around in jungles eating foods that our bodies have been designed to eat in their original form - that you could pluck out of a tree, or pull out of the earth - these foods are likely to be most beneficial for your health. As this diet is mainly based on fresh vegetables, fruits, beans, lentils and wholegrains you will find it very economical. You will need to vary the fruits and vegetables depending on what's in season. Buy the freshest ingredients, organic if possible, since these tend to contain more nutrients.

To help you get started here are some ideas for healthy breakfasts, main meals, salads. Almost all recipes are sugar-free, using the natural sweetness present in food. They are also high in fibre, so you don't need to add any extra. The foods used are naturally high in vitamins and minerals. For snacks choose fruit since many fruits are best digested on their own, together with a few almonds or sunflower seeds.

A few recipes refer to 'sautéeing'. This is quite different from frying. Use a fraction of butter or olive oil, just to lightly coat the saucepan. Warm the oil and add the ingredients. As soon as they are sizzling, add two tablespoons of water or vegetable stock and cook with the lid on. In this way vegetables can be 'steam-fried' using a fraction of the fat used in frying, and taste delicious. Some lunches and dinners give quantities for two or four people. So don't forget to divide the quantities accordingly if you're just cooking for yourself.

BREAKFASTS

Get Up & Go
Get Up & Go is a breakfast drink made by blending skimmed milk or soya milk with a banana and a serving of Get Up & Go. Get Up and Go is a nutrient rich powder containing complex carbohydrates, protein derived from quinoa, vitamins, minerals, sesame, sunflower and pumpkin seeds, oatgerm, oatbran, ricebran and psyllium husks. Each serving provides the RDA of every known essential nutrient, a third of all the protein you need, plus complex carbohydrate, fibre and very little fat. It contains no sucrose, no additives, no animal products, no milk, no wheat and no yeast.

Each serving, with skimmed milk and a banana provides less than 300 calories thus making it ideal as part of a balanced low calorie diet if you need to lose weight. It is available in health food shops (made by Holford's Wholefoods, distributed by Brewhurst.)

1 serving Get Up & Go
1/2 pint (300ml) skimmed milk or soya milk
1 banana
• Blend milk, banana and Get Up & Go powder.

Apple Muesli *(Serves 1)*

Apple Muesli is one of many mueslis you can make yourself. Experiment with other combinations. Apple muesli tastes best soaked overnight in enough water to cover ingredients. Add milk and yoghurt in the morning.

2 tbsp oatflakes or millet flakes; 1 tbsp raisins
1 apple, grated; 2 tbsp natural yoghurt (optional)
1 tbsp (25g) almonds or ground sesame seeds
• Serve with milk or soya milk.

Sesame Porridge *(Serves 1)*

On a cold winter day nothing can be more warming than porridge. Oats contain special factors that are known to promote a healthy heart and arteries and are full of fibre and complex carbohydrates.

1/2 pint (300 ml) water; 1/2 pint (300 ml) skimmed milk or soya milk
1oz (25 g) porridge oats; 1 banana; 1tbsp ground sesame seeds
• Put the water and half the milk in a saucepan and sprinkle in the oats.
• Bring to the boil and boil for five minutes, stirring all the time.
• Serve with a little milk, banana and ground seeds.

Scrambled Egg *(Serves 1)*

While eggs are rather high in fats, as an occasional part of a balanced diet, they are a good source of protein and add variety.

2 free range eggs; 1 tbsp parsley or chives; 1/2 oz (10 g) butter
• Melt butter in a small saucepan. Add beaten eggs and parsley or chives.
• Cook slowly, stirring constantly.
• Serve with whole rye toast.

Fruity Millet Flakes *(Serves 1)*

This satisfying breakfast is a good source of fibre, as well as essential fatty acids.

1 tbsp millet flakes; 1 apple, grated; 1 banana, chopped
Juice of one orange; 1 tbsp (25g) sunflower seeds; Pinch mixed spice
• Soak oats overnight.
• Combine with other ingredients.

Apricot Nut Shake *(Serves 1)*

This is a dairy free alternative to milkshakes.

1 cup water; 2 oz (50 g) almonds; 6 apricots (dried or fresh)
2 tbsp sunflower seeds; 1 tbsp wheatgerm

- If using dried apricots, soak overnight.
- Blend nuts, seeds and water until smooth. Blend in apricots and wheatgerm.

MAIN MEALS

Tofu and Avocado Dip with Crudités *(Serves 2)*

Tofu is an excellent source of protein. This delicous dip allows you to crunch away on a variety of raw vegetables.

4 oz (100 g) tofu; 1/2 ripe avocado; 2 tbsps Quark or soya milk
1 clove garlic; 1 spring onion; 1 tbsp parsley; Pinch paprika
1 tsp tamari or soya sauce; Black pepper

- Blend all the ingredients until smooth.
- Serve with a variety of seasonal crudités - carrots, cucumber, tomato, lettuce, celery, fennel, endive, chinese leaves, mushrooms, peppers, cauliflower or broccoli.

Rice and Bean Sprout Salad *(Serves 2)*

Bean sprouts, being vegetables in their youth, are incredibly rich in nutrients and high in vitality.

4 oz (100 g) brown rice, cooked; 2 tbsp French dressing
4 oz (100 g) bean sprouts; 1 carrot, chopped
1 spring onion, finely sliced

- Pour the dressing over the hot rice and allow it to cool.
- Combine with the other ingredients.

Apple and Tuna Salad *(Serves 2)*

Tuna fish is rich in EFAs.

1 red apple, chopped; 1 small tin tuna fish in brine; 2 sticks celery, sliced
1/3 iceberg lettuce, sliced; 1 handful beansprouts; 1 tbsp mayonnaise
2 tbsp natural yoghurt (optional); Black pepper

- Drain the tuna fish and combine with other salad ingredients.
- Blend the mayonnaise (and yoghurt) and mix in to the salad. Season with black pepper.

Carrot Soup in the Raw *(Serves 4)*

Ever had a hot, raw soup? This soup is made cold and heated gently, keeping all the vitamin and mineral content intact. You can spice it up with Mexican spices or Malaysian curry and a little creamed coconut. Try adding tofu for a thicker soup.

1lb (450 g) carrots; 3 oz (75 g) ground almonds
1/2 pint skimmed milk; 1 tsp vegetable stock; 1 tsp mixed herbs
• Place carrots in a food processor and blend to a puree.
• Add other ingredients and process until mixed.
• Warm very gently in a pan.

Nutty Three Bean Salad *(Serves 1)*

No foods are better than beans for giving stamina.

4 oz (100 g) mixed beans (eg haricots, kidney and flageolet) cooked
A handful of walnuts; Parsley; 1 tbsp French dressing
2 oz (50 g) fennel, chopped; 2 spring onions, finely sliced
• Combine all the ingredients.

Farmhouse Vegetable Soup *(Serves 4)*

Here's a wonderfully warming and easy to make meal in itself.

1.5lb (700 g) chopped fresh seasonal vegetables eg potatoes, swede, celeriac, leeks, celery, carrots, broccoli, cabbage. 1 medium onion; 2 cloves garlic;
1 14oz (450 g) tin tomatoes; 1 tbsp olive oil; 1 tsp vegetable stock
• Sauté the onion and garlic in the oil.
• Add the vegetables, tomatoes, enough water to cover and the vegetable stock.
• Simmer until vegetables are cooked.
This soup can be liquidized or may be left as it is. Use potatoes in moderation as they thicken the soup

Baked Potato, Crudités and Satay Sauce *(Serves 1)*

Potatoes are always unfairly left out of slimming recipes. But do eat the skins since they're full of fibre. When making your own, cook them for as short a time as possible.

1 baked potato; 1 tbsp peanut butter; 1 tbsp tahini
1/2 tbsp lemon juice; 1 clove garlic; A little vegetable stock
• Blend together the sauce ingredients. Serve with the baked potato and a mixture of raw vegetables as crudites.

Mexican Bean Dip and Crudités *(Serves 4)*

This spicy red bean dip is a great accompaniment to raw vegetables.

4 oz (100 g) kidney beans, cooked; 4 oz (100 g) Quark; 1 tbsp olive oil;
1/2 onion, finely chopped; 1 clove garlic, crushed
2 tbsp yoghurt; Pinch chilli powder

• Sauté the onion and garlic gently and add the chilli powder. Cool.
• Blend all the ingredients, adding more yoghurt if necessary to give a smooth creamy dip. Serve with a mixture of raw vegetable crudités.

Hummus *(Serves 4)*

Chick peas, also known as garbanzo beans, have a unique taste which combines well with tahini, a paste of ground sesame seeds. Try sprouting your chick peas first, increasing their vitamin and mineral content. You can also buy hummus ready made.

4 oz (100 g) chick peas, cooked; 1 clove garlic, crushed
1 tbsp olive oil; Juice 1 lemon; 2 tbsp tahini; Cayenne pepper

• Place all the ingredients in a food processor and blend until smooth and creamy, adding extra water if necessary.
• Garnish with a little cayenne pepper.

Carrot Coleslaw *(Serves 4)*

Cabbages are packed with vitamins and minerals. So are carrots, high in vitamin A, and onions, high in sulphur containing amino acids, thought to be good for arthritis.

1 lb (450 g) red or white cabbage; 8 oz (225 g) carrots; 1 small onion
4 oz (100 g) raisins; 2 tbsp low fat mayonnaise; 2 tbsp milk or soya milk

• Finely chop cabbage, carrots and onion.
• Mix all ingredients. Serve with celery and carrot sticks.

Butter Bean and Sweetcorn Soup *(Serves 4)*

This simple soup takes 15 minutes to make.

12 oz (350 g) frozen sweetcorn kernels; 1 oz (25 g) butter
1 clove garlic, crushed; 1 onion, chopped; 2 sticks celery, chopped
4 oz (125 g) butter beans, cooked; 1 pinch thyme
1/2 pint (300 ml) milk or soya milk; 1/2 pint (300 ml) vegetable stock
Black pepper

• Sauté the onion, celery and garlic.
• Add remaining ingredients and simmer for 10 minutes.

Shepherdess Pie (Serves 4)

This vegetarian equivalent of shepherds pie is very tasty.

1 tbsp olive oil; 1 onion, chopped; 1 clove garlic, crushed
14 oz (400 g) tin tomatoes; 12 oz (300 g) aduki beans, cooked
1 tbsp parsley, choppped; 2 tbsp tamari; 1.5lb (700 g) mashed potato 2 oz (50 g) low fat Cheddar cheese, grated (optional)

• Sauté onion and garlic in the oil.
• Add the tomatoes, parsley, aduki beans and tamari. Simmer gently for 15 minutes.
• Place bean mixture in an ovenproof dish and top with mashed potatoes and cheese.
• Bake for 35 minutes at 200C, 400F, gas mark 6.

Sweet and Sour Tofu (Serves 4)

This Chinese style dish has an unusual taste.

1 tbsp olive oil; 1 clove garlic, chopped; 1 onion, chopped
1 green pepper, chopped; 1 carrot, sliced
4 oz (100 g) tinned pineapple chunks (unsweetened); 8 oz (200 g) tofu
Sauce: *2 tsp cornflour; 4 tbsp pineapple juice; 3 tbsp cider vinegar*
1 tbsp brown sugar; 2 tsp soya sauce; 1 tbsp tomato purée

• Sauté the vegetables in the oil.
• Combine the sauce ingredients and add to the vegetables together with the pineapple and tofu. Simmer for three minutes, stirring well.

Chestnut Hotpot (Serves 4)

Chestnuts are the lowest fat nuts by a long way, so enjoy yourself in chestnut season. Out of season you can use dried chestnuts which simply need soaking overnight (and are much easier to prepare!).

5 oz (150 g) dried chestnuts; 1 medium onion, sliced
1 oz (25 g) butter; 8 oz (225 g) parsnip; 8 oz (225 g) potato
8 oz (225 g) swede; 8 oz (225 g) turnip; 1/2 pint vegetable stock
Black pepper

• Soak chestnuts overnight.
• Sauté the onion in the butter.
• Slice all the vegetables and add to the pot with the stock, pepper and chestnuts.
• Simmer very gently until chestnuts are just soft, about 30 - 45 minutes.

Mushroom Pilaf *(Serves 4)*

Mushrooms can be eaten raw in salads, or cooked as in this delicious pilaf. The secret is to cook them slowly. Adding a little water helps to bring out their juices.

8 oz (225 g) brown rice; 1/2 oz butter; I tbsp olive oil; 1 large onion, chopped
1 pint (600 ml) hot water; 2 oz (50 g) raisins; 8 oz (225 g) frozen peas;
8 oz (225 g) mushrooms, sliced; 1 tsp yeast extract;
1 tsp finely chopped root ginger; 2 tbsp parsley, chopped

• Gently heat the oil and butter in a heavy frying pan and fry the rice in it until pale brown. Add onion and cook for a further five minutes.
• Add water, raisins and mushrooms, cover and simmer until liquid is absorbed and rice just tender. Add more hot water if needed.
• Stir in yeast extract and ginger.
• Cook frozen peas, drain and add to rice mixture.
• Serve garnished with parsley.

Spaghetti Napolitana *(Serves 4)*

If you've never tried buckwheat spaghetti this is the recipe to try them with. I prefer buckwheat spaghetti but you have to be a bit careful how you cook it. Bring it to the boil, then add cold water, then bring it back to the boil. Do this twice for best results.

12 oz (300 g) buckwheat spaghetti; 2 medium onions, sliced
2 tbsp olive oil; 3 carrots, chopped; 8 oz (225 g) mushrooms, chopped
I clove garlic, crushed; 1 green pepper, chopped
4 oz (100 g) tomato or carrot purée ; 2 tsp concentrated vegetable stock
1 tsp thyme

• Sauté the onion in the oil.
• Add the vegetables and sauté for 5 minutes.
• Add the vegetable stock, thyme, tomato or carrot purée and enough water to just cover. Simmer for 20 minutes.
• Blend in a food processor.
• Cook the spaghetti in plenty of boiling water for about 12 minutes. Serve topped with the tomato or carrot sauce.

SALADS

Watercress Salad *(Serves 4)*

Watercress is rich in iron and vitamin A and is delicious in salad.

1/2 bunch watercress; 1/3 iceberg lettuce, sliced ; 1/2 cucumber, sliced;
1 green pepper, chopped; 3 handfuls alfalfa sprouts
• Combine all the ingredients and toss with 1 tbsp French dressing

Green Salad *(Serve 4)*

This simple green salad is a good accompaniment to any meal.

1/3 Cos or other lettuce, chopped; 1/4 bulb of fennel, sliced
2 oz (50 g) broccoli tops, chopped; 1/4 cucumber, chopped
2 sticks celery, sliced
• Combine all the ingredients and toss with 1 tbsp French dressing.

Spinach and Bean Salad *(Serves 4)*

Spinach is an underestimated salad food, but care must be taken in preparing the spinach leaves.

1 lb (450 g) fresh spinach; 3 tbsp minced onion
14 oz (350 g) tin kidney beans
For the dressing: *1/2 tbsp olive oil; 1 1/2 tbsp lemon juice*
1/2 tsp bouillion powder
• Strip the spinach leaves from the stalk and soak in a tub of cold water.
• Lift leaves and rinse under running water.
• Drain and pat dry.
• Chop the leaves and toss with the onions and half the beans.
• Arrange the rest of the beans on top.
• Mix the dressing ingredients together and pour over the salad.

Garden Salad with Avocado Dressing

• Mix lettuce, tomato, spring onion, brocolli, mangetout, courgette and herbs.
For the dressing
• Puree the avocado with a little lemon juice, a clove of garlic and some vegetable stock.

25

Supplementary Benefit

Whatever view you may have about supplements the reality is that you can achieve far better results with arthritis with the judicial use of supplements plus diet, than with diet alone. Vitamins and minerals are considerably less toxic than drugs and are unlikely to have anything other than positive effects, provided you stick within the guidelines of this book. Many arthritis sufferers have reversed their condition and remained drug-free through the combination of diet, supplements, exercise and postural alignment.

Vitamins and Minerals

The best place to start with a supplement programme is to take a good all-round multivitamin and mineral programme since nutrients work together. The basic intake I recommend for each nutrient is shown in the Figure 19 on page 135 as the Basic Level. This is the level to supplement on top of a good diet, assuming you will be following the dietary guidelines in this book. This basic level equates to, for example, a multivitamin, a multimineral and 3 vitamin C 1,000mg tablets. It may cost you 35p a day - the price of a bar of chocolate, a bag of crisps, a cup of coffee, a fraction of a glass of wine or pint of beer, or three cigarettes. If you show this chart to a health food shop assistant they should be able to find the easiest and cheapest way to meet these levels. On page 154 you'll find a list of good supplements and brands to choose from.

Essential Fatty Acids

The next additional extras are the essential fatty acids GLA and EPA. These are not strictly speaking essential since GLA can be derived from linoleic acid, and EPA from linolenic acid, both of which are rich in seeds and their oil. So, if you are eating enough of these you may not 'need' to supplement extra GLA or EPA. However, both have been shown to help reduce inflammation and are well worth experimenting with. Often, the best way to do this is to start with the maximum therapeutic level for one month, then, if that helps, reduce to the basic level and see if the improvement remains. GLA is found in evening primrose oil and borage oil. 500mg of evening primrose oil provides around 50mg of GLA. So the basic level is 3 capsules of 500mg evening primrose oil a day.

EPA and DHA are found together in fish oil. A capsule of fish oil providing EPA is almost certain to provide DHA in the right proportion, so EPA and DHA come together. 3,000mg of fish oil will give you around 1,000mg of EPA. Again, start with the maximum therapeutic dose, then, if this helps, reduce to the basic level after a month. You can also experiment with increasing oily fish in your diet.

Both EHA and GLA supplements are relatively expensive, however they are prescribable by your GP. If you find they help it is well worth discussing this with your doctor to see if you can continue to get your supplies by prescription.

The Therapeutic Use of Vitamins and Minerals

You may then wish to experiment with increasing the intake of some nutrients which have been shown to have particularly beneficial effects on certain types of arthritis. I recommend starting with vitamin B3 and B5. Both have proven effective in all kinds of arthritis and both are relatively inexpensive. Try these individually for two months at the maximum therapeutic level. If this helps try reducing the dose and see if the benefit is maintained. If not return to the higher dose. If there is no change in the two months then return to the basic dose.

The next experiment to try, especially if you have rheumatoid arthritis or inflammatory problems, is increasing the levels of anti-oxidant nutrients selenium, vitamins C and E. Once again increase your intake of these nutrients to the maximum therapeutic levels for one month. (If you get loose bowels on so much vitamin C reduce your intake accordingly.) If this makes a difference gradually lower the doses until you find the lowest level that maintains the benefit.

You can also experiment with increasing your intake of the other important minerals including calcium, magnesium, zinc, iron, copper, manganese and chromium. This can be done by taking an extra multimineral. In truth, it is best to have a mineral test, such as a hair mineral analysis, in case you may already have high levels of copper and iron, both of which can be harmful.

Optional Extras

Finally, there are optional extras you may like to try. These include the amino acid DLPA for pain control, and mussel extract, shark cartilage or s-adenosyl-methionine, all of which provide vital building material for cartilage. Start with the maximum therapeutic level for one month. If this has a positve effect reduce to the basic level and see if the improvement continues.

Safety First

All the levels of nutrients I have recommended fall well below the lowest levels at which adverse or toxic reactions have been reported. Please do not exceed the maximum therapeutic levels unless under the guidance of a qualified nutrition consultant or doctor. You may wisely choose to carry out these experiments under the guidance of a qualified nutritionist (see page 158 to find one in your area). They can often speed up the process of helping you find the most effective supplement regime. If, in any event, you experience either severe adverse reactions, or minor adverse reactions that persist for more than three days stop taking whatever you suspect of causing these reactions and consult a qualified nutrition consultant or your doctor.

Knowing What Works

To find out what works for you it is best to experiment with the mind of a scientist. In other words change one thing at a time, give it long enough to have an effect, and monitor changes. For most nutrients one month is the shortest time and two months the longest time you need to know if something is likely to help you.

Once you've been on your basic vitamin and mineral programme add one extra item at a time so you know what makes a difference. If a nutrient makes a difference add this to your basic programme and then experiment with something else. Don't keep taking 'maximum therapeutic levels' of something that shows no clear result.

Nutrient	Basic Level	Max. Therapeutic Level
Vitamins		
A - beta-carotene	7,500iu	-
C - ascorbic acid	3,000mg	10,000mg
E - d-alpha tocopherol	400iu	600iu
D - cholecalciferol (D3)	400iu	
B1 - thiamine	25mg	
B2 - riboflavin	25mg	
B3 - niacinamide	50mg	1,000mg
B5 - pantothenic acid	50mg	1,000mg
B6 - pyridoxine	50mg	
B12 - cyanocobalamine	10mcg	
Folic Acid	100mcg	
Biotin	50mcg	
Minerals		
Calcium	300mg	600mg
Magnesium	300mg	600mg
Iron	10mg	
Zinc	10mg	35mg
Copper	1mg	3mg
Manganese	2.5mg	25mg
Selenium	100mcg	200mcg
Chromium	50mcg	200mcg
Essential Fatty Acids		
GLA	150mg	300mg
EPA	1,200mg	1,800mg
DHA	800mg	1,200mg
Amino Acids & Other Nutrients		
DLPA		750mg
Mussel Extract	250mg	1,000mg
Shark Cartilage Extract	1,000mg	10,000mg
S-Adenosyl-Methionine	1,000mg	5,000mg

Figure 19 Optimum Supplemental Intakes of Nutrients for Arthritis

Chapter 29 explains how to monitor your improvement and keep a good record on your experiments with these different nutrients. These records will help any practitioner you may consult at a later date, so don't throw them away.

When To Take Supplements

Vitamins, minerals, essential fatty acids and amino acids all work together in the body and are designed to be taken in together. So it is best to take additional supplements of nutrients with food. The enzymes produced in the digestive tract also help to break down the protein coating on some supplements. You can split the supplements you take over the meals in the day. However if taking supplements twice a day would mean that you'd forget the second lot it is probably best to take them all at once. Here are the 'ten commandments' of supplement taking:

1 Take vitamins and minerals 15 minutes before or after, or during a meal.

2 Take most of your supplements with your first meal of the day.

3 Don't take B vitamins late at night if you have difficulty sleeping.

4 Take multivitamins or dolomite tablets in the evening - these help you sleep.

5 If you're taking two or more B Complex or vitamin C tablets take one at each meal.

6 Don't take individual B vitamins unless you are also taking a general B Complex, perhaps in a multivitamin.

7 Don't take individual minerals unless you are also taking a general multivitamin.

8 If you are anaemic (iron deficient) take extra iron with vitamin C. Avoid 'ferric' forms of iron.

9 If you know you are copper deficient take copper only with 10 times as much zinc, e.g. 0.5mg copper to 5mg zinc.

10 Always take your supplements every day. Irregular supplementation doesn't work.

26

Identifying and Eliminating Allergies

Not everyone who has arthritis is allergic or sensitive to certain foods. So how do you know if you are?

Are You Allergic?

If you get three or more of these symptoms, as well as joint or muscle aches, there is a good chance that you might be.

Hay-fever, a stuffy and running nose, itchy eyes, itchy skin, asthma or difficulty breathing, headaches, bloating, water retention, facial puffiness, discolouration around the eyes.

If you eat any one of these foods most days and would find them difficult to give up, it's worth testing to see if you're allergic to them.

Wheat (bread, biscuits, cereals), dairy produce (milk, cheese, yoghurt), meat, alcohol (especially beer and wine), coffee, chocolate, peanuts, eggs, oranges.

How to Test for Allergies

Avoid all the substances you suspect, whether within the above list or not, strictly for 20 days. If you have completed the 10 Day Detox Diet then you only have ten days to go. Do check the contents of the foods you eat carefully to see whether they contain any of the above. It is best to prepare yourself well by stocking up with your allergen free foods before starting.

If you are avoiding WHEAT stay off all bread, cakes, biscuits, pasta, sauces, cereals etc. Alternatives are oat cakes, rice cakes, genuine 100% rye bread such as pumpernickel or volkenbrot, rye crispbread, sauces made with corn flour, corn or oat based cereals and pastry made with corn and almond meal instead of wheat.

If you are avoiding all GRAINS stay off anything containing wheat, rye, oats, barley, corn or spelt (an ancient wheat strain). You can eat rice, millet, buckwheat or quinoa. Reintroduce foods starting with corn, then oats, barley, spelt, rye then wheat.

If you are avoiding MILK stay off all milk, cheese, yoghurt, butter, chocolate and foods containing milk produce. Good alternatives are soya milk, or nut cream, made by blending nuts with water (cashews are particularly good). Drink herb teas that do not require milk, and have more free range eggs if cheese is a major source for your protein.

If you are avoiding YEAST stay off all yeasted breads, spreads, and beer. Be very careful to check the label, on baked products.

Then Do This Simple Pulse Test

1 Take your pulse at rest (after five minutes sitting down), for 60 seconds. Your pulse can be found inside the boney protruberance on the thumb side of your wrist.
2 Then eat more than usual of the No. 1 food.
3 Take your pulse after 10, 30 and 60 minutes. Make sure you take your pulse at rest for the duration of 60 seconds.
4 Keep a record of any symptoms over the next 24 hours.

If your pulse increases by 10 points or if you have any noticeable symptoms within 24 hours, avoid this substance and wait 48 hours before testing the next item on your list.

If your pulse does not increase by 10 points *and* you have no change in symptoms, reintroduce this food (in moderation) into your diet, and proceed with the same test for food No.2.

Continue in this way for other suspected substances.

If you've ever had severe allergic reactions, and or an attack of asthma, this test should not be carried out without the supervision of a doctor or nutritionist.

This method of testing for allergies is not fool proof, especially if you have delayed reactions to foods. However it is a very good place to start and is often as effective as expensive tests. If you do suspect you have allergies yet cannot clearly identify them with this method then it is best to consult an allergy specialist.

27
Reducing Stress

We all need some stimulation or we decline into apathy. Indeed, boredom can also be a stress. For many of us overstimulation, leading to excessive stress, is the problem. Since we all have different abilities for coping with different circumstances each person has an optimal stress level.

In order to avoid excessive stress it is important to understand the signs and symptoms of stress, and its causes. Stress - anger, fear, excitement, frustration - stimulates the adrenal glands. So do certain chemical substances, including refined sugar, salt, cigarettes, alcohol, tea and coffee. All these things, in excess, cause the same reaction.

What Stress Does

The stress reaction is a physical one, for the very good reason that when primitive man had feelings of stress, the cause was likely to be physical danger. His body reactions prepared him to run away fast, or to turn and fight.

The adrenal glands therefore release adrenalin, which produces a 'high' almost like a drug. They also release cortisone. Together, these two hormones gear the whole body for action. Digestion shuts down. Glucose is released into the bloodstream to fuel the nerves and muscles. Breathing, heart rate and blood pressure all increase, ready to deliver oxygen to the cells to burn the fuel and make energy.

Too Much Stress

If this process happens too often, side effects build up. Nutrients are used up. Digestion is slow and disrupted. Resistance to infection declines. Minor problems build up, such as headaches, stiffness, insomnia or moodiness. If nothing is done, major problems can occur, such as heart disease, diabetes, arthritis and even cancer.

The adrenal glands can become exhausted from over-stimulation. So can the thyroid, which works closely with the adrenals. More and more stimulation is needed to get them working, so there maybe cravings for harmful stimulants like sugar and coffee. As the systems become worn down, there may be weight gain, higher blood cholesterol, slower thinking and reduced energy.

Action Against Stress

In most stress situations, the most we do is drum our fingers or make a rude remark, or even worse, keep our feelings bottled up inside, leading to hidden resentment. This is not enough to use up the nutrients released into the blood and the physical mechanisms designed to burn them up.

This is why exercise is important for people who are stressed in any way. Obviously it is best taken at the time of stress - a brisk walk or vigorous exercise session is good first-aid for feelings of stress. If that is impossible, you will benefit from regular exercise.

Simple relaxation techniques also help the body and mind to get back to normal. Tense your muscles as hard as you can and then relax, starting with your feet and ending with your facial muscles. Or just clench your fists tightly and relax. Or take a deep breath, hold it for a count of 10, and breathe it all out at once. Yoga breathing or meditation exercises are excellent de-stressors.

Long-Term Stress Control

Your real need, however, is to counter stress at source. Try these suggestions:

- limit your working hours to, at most, 10 hours a day, five days a week.
- keep at least 1.5 days a week completely free of routine work.
- make sure you use this free time to cultivate a relaxing hobby, do something creative or take exercise, preferably in the fresh air.
- adopt a relaxed manner. For instance, walk and talk more slowly. A useful idea is to act 'as if' you were a relaxed person, almost as a game.
- avoid obvious pressures, such as taking on too many commitments. learn to say 'no', or 'not for now'.

- learn to see when a problem is somebody else's responsibility and refuse to take it on.
- if you have an emotional problem you cannot solve alone, seek advice.
- concentrate on one task at a time, and focus all your attention on the present.
- learn to say what is on your mind instead of suppressing it. You don't have to be aggressive - just to state your point of view clearly and truthfully.
- listen to what other people say to you, and about you.
- look long and hard at all the stresses in your life. Make a list of them. Set out to find a positive attitude to things which can't be changed. If change is possible - take action. Don't let things wear you down.

28

Your Hydrotherapy and Exercise Programme

Exercise and hydrotherapy is a vital part of any anti-arthritis programme. The key is setting yourself a realistic routine and sticking to it. For the first few weeks you may need to exercise your will as well as your body, but once established exercise becomes a habit that is as hard to break as not exercising. Establish a routine that works for you, given your lifestyle. However, the following routine provides a good basis for you to adapt. Monitor your progress as explained in Chapter 29.

DAY 1 & 4

Warm Up
Neck
Arms
Hands
Back
Knees
Feet
Cool Down

Shower - Hot & Cold - before and/or after exercise session

These are your suppleness and strength exercise days. Make sure, over the two days, you exercise all these areas and their related joints. Exercise arthritic or achey joints in both sessions. Initially, aim for 15 minutes. Then build this to 30 to 60 minutes. These exercises are generally best done in the morning or evening. Start each session with warm up exercises to relax, lengthen and bring circulation to the muscles you are about to work.

Another great way to do this is to start with a warm shower, then turn the tap to cold. Shower each area of your body that is affected, rubbing the area with your hands and mentally becoming conscious of this area, saying inwardly "I bring consciousness to my knees etc.". The cold water brings energy to the joint which responds with a warm glow. Follow this with your warm up exercises.

DAY 2 & 6

Aerobic Exercise

Alkalising Bath

These days are for building your stamina through aerobic exercise. By definition aerobic exercise needs to be hard work and get your heart beating faster. Good examples are swimming, walking, bicycling, stair-climbing, exercise or dance classes. Whatever you choose make sure the exercise is low impact and doesn't overstrain your joints. Invest in a good pair of shoes and don't overstretch yourself. Aim for 15 minutes to start with, then build up to 30 to 60 minutes depending on the kind of exercise. Swimming for 15 minutes, for example, is equivalent to more than half an hour brisk walking. A good routine is to swim once a week and walk once a week. As with days 1 and 3 start each session with warm up exercises and end each session with cool down exercises.

After each aerobic exercise session have a soothing warm bath adding 100g of sodium bicarbonate which you can buy in any chemist. Acid by-products are produced when muscles work hard. Sodium bicarbonate has an alkalising effect and reduces muscle stiffness.

DAY 3 & 7

Massage & Relaxation

If you can it is well worth having a therapeutic massage once a week or once a fortnight. This can help to improve healing and circulation, as well as helping to relax traumatised muscles. Alternatively, learn how to give yourself a massage. Self-massage is the highest form of healing since it is you directing your will to heal yourself. Some areas of the body, however, are rather hard to reach. It is a good idea to have an alkalising bath after such a massage as well.

Leave one day a week completely free of any routine. Relax and enjoy yourself.

The Exercises

When you see a physical health professional they can recommend specific exercises for you to carry out. Exercises for each body area are also given in a number of excellent books that focus precisely on this area. The two I particularly recommend are Exercise Beats Arthritis by Valerie Sayce and Ian Fraser, and Office Yoga by Julie Friedberger (see Recommended Reading on page 151).

A Word of Caution

If a joint is aching or inflammed either perform very light, loosening exercises that take the joint through its range of motion, or rest the joint completely. Make sure you do not overstress any aching joint. Know your body's limit and do not cause yourself unnecessary pain. This will slow down your healing, not speed it up. Use cold compresses to calm down a hot, inflamed joint.

29
Monitoring Your Progress

Monitoring your progess in a systematic way has two advantages. The first is that you are more likely to find out what makes a difference to your arthritis. Too often people embark on a new regime which contains some pieces of advice that help them and others that do not. For example, a diet that excludes all common allergens may help, but unless you investigate how you feel with or without specific foods you may end up eating an unnecessarily restrictive diet. The second advantage of monitoring is that it helps you to stick to the regime you wish to follow.

Monitoring Change

The first step to monitoring is to pick specific symptoms that can change. This may be pain, joint flexibility, morning stiffness, swelling or general lack of energy. I suggest you pick three or four symptoms your can genuinely rate as 'better' or 'worse' from week to week. Take one of these, for example 'pain'. If you have no pain give that a Health Rating of 100%. If you have unbearable pain give that a Health Rating of 0%. What is the worst you've ever been? Where are you now?

Pick a time, perhaps on Sunday, when you can look back over the week and assess whether your pain has been worse or better. (You may be able to assess this by keeping a record of how often you use pain-killing drugs, if you do.) If you started at 30% and have improved a little rate yourself 40%. Next Sunday assess whether your pain level is better, the same, or worse. Do this for each of your symptoms, using a different coloured pen for each symptom, week by week. This gives you a yardstick to see what makes a difference. Make a note of which symptom is in which colour on your Monitoring Progress Chart.

Setting Your Target

Be realistic in the targets you set. Take it one step at a time. Set yourself targets for changing your diet and taking exercise that you know you will reach. It is far better to take one step towards permanently changing your lifestyle, than to take four steps back, on an over-ambitious regime.

So decide what you are going to do for the next month ahead. Be realistic and specific,write it down and stick it up somewhere you can see it. This, plus weekly monitoring, will remind you to keep on track. Be patient with yourself. Big changes to diet and lifestyle, which I believe are your best chance of conquering arthritis, happen by a series of small changes. If you've had pain for five years if may take you one year to find your best regime. The effects of exercise, diet and supplements are not as rapid as drugs, but they are accumulative. Once your diet and lifestyle has changed for the better, and you feel better, it is very hard to go back to old habits.

Record Changes in Treatment and Compliance

Whenever you change your treatment make a note of this. For example, if you decide to experiment with B3 (niacinamide) 1,000mg for a month write this down in week 4. If your doctor lowers the dose of your medication note this too. If you decide to avoid alcohol for a month put this down as well. It is best not to make too many changes at once so you can see what is making a difference.

At the end of each week rate yourself on your compliance to the targets you've set yourself for diet, supplements and exercise (this could be physical exercise, hydrotherapy or/and postural exercises).

* * * * means you met your targets. Well done.
* * *   means you more or less stuck to your targets. Good.
* *   means you only stuck to your targets half-heartedly.
*   means you went off the rails and didn't stick to your targets.

Notice what difference your level of compliance makes to your health rating. Start every week anew. If you didn't do well last

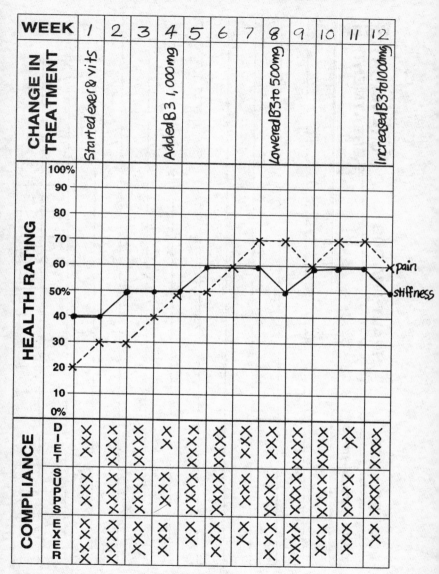

Figure 20 Example Monitoring Progress Chart

147

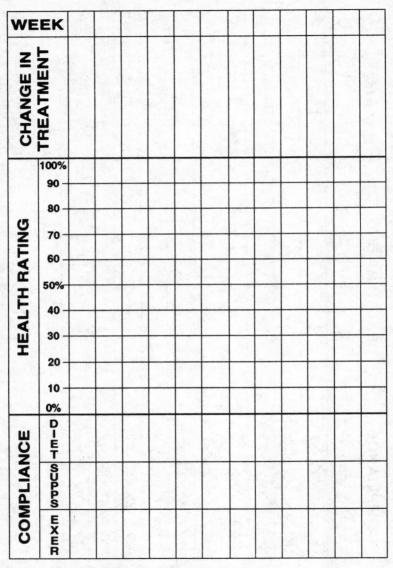

Figure 21 *Monitoring Progress Chart*

© Patrick Holford   You have the permission of the author and publisher to photocopy this chart for your own personal use only.

week, that's history. This week do your best to stick to your chosen goal.

On page 147 you'll see an example of a completed Monitoring Progress Chart over a 12 week period. You write in the weeks so that you can photocopy the blank Monitoring Progress Chart on page 148 and use this for the months that follow. Don't throw these charts away. Should you consult a health practitioner these can help them to see, at a glance, how you've been getting on.

Arthritis Research at ION

At the Institute for Optimum Nutrition in London, where I practice and teach, we are often conducting research into new approaches for arthritis. If you'd like to take part in this research send an SAE to me addressed ARTHRITIS RESEARCH c/o ION, 5 Jerdan Place, London SW6 1BE. We are also collecting information from people like yourself, who've tried different strategies to assess whether they work or not, and for whom they are best suited. We'd love to hear from you and would ask you to send copies of your Monitoring Progress Chart, plus a brief history of your illness. Many thanks for any help you can give us in this on-going research and I wish you great success in saying NO to arthritis.

Other Natural Remedies from Devil's Claw to Yucca

Yucca

A double-blind trial found that an extract of saponin, from the Yucca plant, benefitted arthritis sufferers [1]. The onset of improvement was gradual and the suggestion was that the extract was indirectly helping the joints, perhaps through effects on bacteria in the gut. The wrong bacteria in the gut can inhibit production of mucopolysaccharides, so essential for joints, so this is a possibility. If this proves to be the case other saponin rich herbs may prove to be of benefit.

Devil's Claw

Devil's Claw (*harpagophytum procumbens*) may be one such herb, being a rich source of saponins. One animal study reported anti-inflammatory effects from this herb [2], while others have not [3]. At this stage the evidence is not conclusive.

Quercetin

Quercetin is a naturally occurring bioflavanoid that is likely to feature in the future treatment of inflammatory diseases. Bioflavanoids are frequently found in nature along with vitamin C. Quercetin is a non-citrus bioflavanoid found in onions, broccoli, squash and red grapes. While I am unaware of any trials yet conducted on arthritis all the evidence on quercetin's effects on the body's biochemistry are encouraging. It has been shown to inhibit the production of the pro-inflammatory prostaglandins (type 2) [4]. Quercetin also inhibits the release of histamine which are involved in inflammatory reactions, and helps to stabilise cells, reduce collagen breakdown and free radical activity all of which are the markers of a good anti-inflammatory agent for arthritis [5-8]. Quercetin is available in health food stores and is probably worth experimenting with in doses of 500mg per day, taken between meals. There is a suggestion, however, that quercetin, in large amounts, may lower body levels of oestrogen. Therefore caution is urged for women of 40 and more.

Recommended Reading

Optimum Nutrition, *Patrick Holford*, ION Press, 1992, £4.95. This book defines optimum nutrition and how to achieve it. It contains a step-by-step plan to work out your own diet and supplement programme.

Optimum Nutrition Workbook, *Patrick Holford*, ION Press, 1992, £9.95. This 209 page, large format book is packed with informative diagrams and covers all the facts about nutrition and is the sequel to *Optimum Nutrition*.

Exercise That Beats Arthritis, *Valerie Sayce and Ian Fraser*, Thorsons, 1991, £9.99. This large format book contains a comprehensive, easy-to-follow programme of exercises.

Office Yoga, *Julie Friedberger*, Thorsons, 1991, £5.95. This survival handbook for the deskbound contains excellent exercises for arthritis sufferers.

How to Boost Your Immune System, *Jennifer Meek*, ION Press, 1988, £2.50. How the immune system works and how to boost it for relief from infections, allergies and immune diseases.

How to Improve Your Digestion and Absorption, *Christopher Scarfe*, ION Press, 1990, £2.50. A practical guide to improving the many problems of a poorly functioning digestive system.

References

Over 160 references from respected scientific literature have been referred to in this book. A full list of these references, listed in sequential order with the numbers corresponding to the subscript numbers in the text, is available from the Institute for Optimum Nutrition, 5 Jerdan Place, London, SW6 1BE. Please send a large SAE.

Glossary

Angiogenesis is the process whereby tissue in the body develops a blood supply *(vascularisation)*.

Ankylosis spondylitis is an inflammatory disease of the lower spine and sacroiliac joint whereby ligaments become inflammed and vertebrae begin to fuse together.

Arachidonic acid is a fatty acid that can lead to the formation of inflammatory prostaglandins.

Arthrosis is a degenerative disease of joints without inflammation.

Arthritis is a degenerative disease of joints involving inflammation.

Bursa is a protective, fluid-filled cushion between bones and muscles designed to protect muscles and ligaments from chaffing.

Bursitis is inflammation of a bursa.

Calcitonin is a hormone produced in the thyroid gland that helps to maintain calcium balance.

Calcitriol is a hormone derived from vitamin D that helps to control calcium balance.

Cartilage is a hard material, softer than bone, that is found at bone ends and between verterbrae, as well as in other parts of the body. It is made from a protein-carbohydrate complex containing mucopolysaccharides.

Chondrocyte is a cell that produces cartilage.

Cortisol is a type of corticosteroid that is given as a drug. Corticosteroid is a fat-based hormone produced by the adrenal cortex that influences blood sugar balance and inflammatory processes, among other effects.

DGLA *(di-homo-gamma-linolenic-acid)* is a fatty acid that is made in the body from linoleic acid. It is a precursor for prostaglandins.

DHA *(docosahexaenoic acid)* is a fatty acid found in fish, made from linolenic acid. It is a precursor for anti-inflammatory prostaglandins.

DLPA *(dl-phenylalanine)* is an amino acid that may relieve pain.

EHA *(eicosapentaenoic acid)* is a fatty acid found in fish, made from linolenic acid. It is a precursor for anti-inflammatory prostaglandins.

ESR is a measure of erythrocyte (red blood cell) sedimentation rate and, when raised, reflects a general state of inflammation.

Leukotrienes are similar to prostaglandins.

Mucopolysaccharides are a key component of cartilage. Polysaccharide is a complex carbohydrate, made of simple carbohydrate units *(sugar)* strung together.

NSAID is a non-steroidal anti-inflammatory drug.

Oestrogen is a hormone produced in the ovaries that regulates the female sexual cycle. Oestrogen levels effect the uptake and utilisation of calcium in the body.

Osteoathritis is a degenerative disease of joints initially involving cartilage and bone degeneration which leads to inflammation.

Osteophyte is a boney spur that can form on the edge of a joint.

Osteoporosis is a disease where the bones become increasingly porous and more likely to fracture.

Parathormone is a hormone produced by the parathyroid gland that helps to control calcium balance by encouraging calcium to go from bone to blood.

Parathyroid glands are four glands that produce parathormone, located behind the thyroid gland at the base of the throat.

Phenylalanine is an essential amino acid.

Polymyalgia means multiple or systemic muscle pain and is a common syndrome found particularly in older women.

Prostaglandins are short-lived substances that control many vital body processes, including inflammation, somewhat like hormones.

Proteoglycans is a type of mucopolysaccharide.

Spondylosis is a condition where there is spinal fusion but no inflammation.

Synovial membrane surrounds the joint space enclosing the synovial fluid.

Synovial fluid is a lubricating liquid produced in synovial cells and secreted into the joint space to lubricate the joint.

Tendonitis is inflammation of a tendon where it attaches to bone.

Tenosynovitis is inflammation of the sheath surrounding a tendon.

Tinnitus is ringing in the ears.

Thyroid gland is a gland at the base of the throat that produces thyroxin, a hormone that helps to control the rate of metabolism, and calcitonin, a hormone that helps to control calcium balance.

Directory of Supplement Companies

Bio Care produce a wide range of supplements available by mail-order. These include Mega GLA Complex, Emulsified Linseed Oil, Efaplex which is Linseed Oil and GLA in combination, Amino-Plex combining sulphur containing amino acids including methionine, anti-oxidant nutrients individually and in combination, calcium and magnesium individually and in combination. Their best multivitamin is Multi Vitamin/Mineral Complex. Send for a free catalogue to: *Bio Care, 54 Northfield Road, Kings Norton, Birmingham, B30 1JH Tel: 021 433 3727.*

Cantassium produce their own high quality vitamins and minerals, available through health food shops and by mail order. Their best multivitamin is *Cantamega 2000*. Their range includes Pantothenic Acid 500mg (Cantopal), Evening Primrose Oil, EPA/DHA, Green Lipped Mussel Extract, Amino acids including DLPA and Methionine, Antioxidants - individually and in combination, Vitamin C and a range of good, high potency all round multivitamins and minerals. Mail order catalogues free from: *Cantassium, 225 Putney Bridge Road, London SW15 2PY Tel: 081 874 1130/5631.*

Green Farm supply the high quality *Natural Flow* and exceptional *Nature's Plus* range of supplements. Their best multivitamin is *Natural Flow Mega Multi*. Their range includes Niacinamide 500mg, Pantothenic acid 500mg, Evening Primrose Oil, EPA/DHA, Amino acids, Antioxidants individually and in combination, Calcium, Magnesium, Vitamin D, Boron, Vitamin C and a range of high potency all round vitamins and minerals. Available through health food shops and by mail order. Free catalogues from:*Green Farm Catalogue, 225 Putney Bridge Road, London SW15 2PY Tel: 081 874 1130/5631.*

Health+Plus produce an extensive range of supplements available by mail order including the *VV Pack,* a good all round multivitamin and mineral, Evening Primrose Oil 500mg, EPA 1,000mg, Supercholine providing 250mg of Pantothenic Acid, and anti-oxidant nutrients individually and together in New Immunade containing vitamin A,C,E, selenium, zinc, calcium and magnesium.Send for a free catalogue to: *Health+Plus Ltd, PO Box 86, Seaford, East Sussex BN25 4ZW Tel: 0323 492096.*

Nature's Best produce an extensive range of supplements available by mail order. Their best multivitamin and mineral is *Multi-Guard.* Other products include Nicotinamide (niacinamide) 100mg, Pantothenic Acid 500mg - time release, Evening Primrose Oil, EPA/DHA, Seatone - Green Lipped Mussel extract, DLPA complex, L-Methionine, Calcium, Magnesium and Boron combinations, and anti-oxidant nutrients. Write or phone for a free 76 page colour catalogue to: *Nature's Best Health Products Ltd, Freepost, Tunbridge Wells TN2 3BR Tel: 0892 534143 (orders)/539595(nutrition advice).*

Quest produce an extensive range of high quality supplements available through health food shops. Their best multivitamin is *Super-Once-A-Day.* Other products include Pantothenic Acid 250mg, Gammaoil 1000 (GLA 100mg), DLPA, Calcium, Magnesium and Boron individually and in combination, and anti-oxidant vitamins A, C, E and selenium. In case of difficulty contact: *Quest Vitamins Ltd, 1 Premier Trading Estate, Dartmouth, Middleway, Birmingham B7 4AT Tel:021 359 0056.*

Solgar produce an extensive range of supplements available through health food shops. These include DLPA 500mg, L-Methionine 500mg, Niacinamide 550mg, Pantothenic Acid 550mg, anti-oxidant nutrients individually and in combination in the Advanced Antioxidant Formula, Calcium, Magnesium and Boron in combination, GLA, EPA, Cartilade and Quercetin. Their best multivitamin supplement is *VM2000* or *VM75.* For your nearest stockist contact: *Solgar Vitamins, Solgar House, Chiltern Commerce Centre, Asheridge Road, Chesham, Bucks HP5 2PY Tel:0494 791691.*

Index

Useful Addresses

The Nutrition Consultants Association publish a directory of nutrition consultants trained at ION (price £1.50) which is available direct from ION.

The Institute for Optimum Nutrition 5 Jerdan Place, London SW6 1BE Tel: 071 385 7984 offers courses and personal consultations with qualified nutrition consultants including Patrick Holford. On request ION will send you a free information pack. See overleaf.

The Osteopathic Information Service 37, Soho Square, London W1V 5DG Tel: 071 439 7177 supply free information on osteopathy including how to find an osteopath in your area.

The Institute of Pure Chiropractic 14 Park End Street, Oxford OX1 1HH Tel: 0865 246687 will supply a directory of chiropractors on request.

The British Chiropractic Association 29 Whitley Street, Reading, Berks RG2 0EG Tel: 0734 757557 will supply a directory of chiropractors for £1, or give you the name of practitioners in your area by phone.

The Society of Teachers of the Alexander Technique (STAT) 20, London House, 266 Fulham Road, London SW10 9EL Tel: 071-351 0828. They'll send you a free directory if you send a stamped addressed envelope.

FSL Unit 1, Riverside Business Centre, Victoria Street, High Wycombe, Bucks HP11 2LT Tel: 0494 448727 supply a wide range of full spectrum lighting including bulbs and tubes.

Pelvic Posture Ltd Oaklands, New Mill Lane, Eversley, Hants RG27 0RA Tel: 0734 732365 supply a wide range of chairs and pelvic support accesories to encourage good posture.

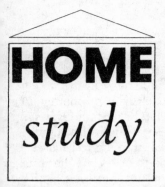

HOME
study

Your car comes with a manual, but what about your body? Do you ever wonder what makes you tick? How you make energy from food? Why some people age faster than others? How to stay super healthy?

You'll find the answers in ION's Homestudy Course (that comes with 3 workbooks, 3 hours of video presentations, 12 taped lectures and step by step instructions to give you a solid grounding in optimum nutrition in 10 weeks.)

You'll learn more about nutrition than you thought possible - and have fun doing it, with practical homework, video presentations and taped lectures. The lecturers include many world authorities in nutrition. For example Professor Bryce-Smith will teach you how to protect yourself from pollution, Patrick Holford shows you how to promote vitality with vitamins and minerals, and Dr. Carl Pfeiffer teaches you how to prevent depression and improve memory.

Part 1 HOW YOUR BODY WORKS, teaches you how to improve digestion and absorption; balance nerves and hormones; and boost immune power. The second part, FOOD AND NUTRITION, looks at everything from the politics of food to wholefood cookery. You'll find out how to prevent heart disease and protect against cancer and arthritis, as well as learning how to detect your own allergies. In the final part, INDIVIDUAL NUTRITION, you'll learn how to work out individually tailored programmes. You'll find out all about nutrition for children and the elderly, as well as how to use nutrition for "first aid".

By the end of the course you'll know enough about nutrition to keep yourself and your family healthy. And you'll be able to help and advise your friends too.

When you enrol for the course you'll get all the course materials including the tapes, videos and workbooks which include written and practical homework for each section of the course.

The course costs less than £10 a week, including all course material. Anyone can do it. All you need is a keen interest in nutrition.

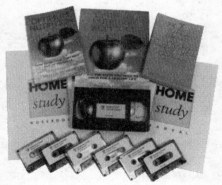

A DETAILED PROSPECTUS IS AVAILABLE ON REQUEST

I. O. N.

The Institute for Optimum Nutrition is a non profit-making independent organisation that exists to help you promote your health through nutrition. ION was founded in 1984 and is based in London. ION offers educational courses starting with a one-day introductory course right up to a two year training to become a nutrition consultant; a clinic for one-to-one consultations; publications; and ION's magazine, Optimum Nutrition, which goes out free to members. If you'd like to receive more details please complete the details below.

Please send me your:

☐ FREE Information Pack
☐ Homestudy Course prospectus
☐ ION Clinic details
☐ Directory of Nutrition Consultants (enclose £1.50)

I'd like to order the following books: *(please list title, quantity & price)*

_____

_____

_____

I enclose £_____ payable to ION *(Please add 10% for p&p)*

First Name: _____ Surname: _____

Address: _____

_____

_____ Post Code: _____

Now send this to: ION, 5 Jerdan Place, London, SW6 1BE
(Tel: 071-385 7984)